Victoria's 95 Secrets
TO A HAPPY, HEALTHY, LONG LIFE

BY 95-YEAR-YOUNG
victoria d. schmidt

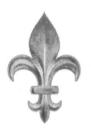

Symbol of Purity
and the
Divine Right To Living

-Dedication-

*I dedicate this book
to my husband **Ralph** and our daughter **Lisa***

Special note: ¬ The "secrets" offered in this book have been researched and are subject to change. It is imperative that they be practiced only after consulting with a physician or a qualified health professional to ensure you are physically fit to undertake them.

Cover Art and Graphic Design: Edward Coutain
Editors: Elizabeth Cody Kimmel and Kevin Anderson

Published by Antigone Press, LLC

Victoria's 95 Secrets
Copyright 2016 by Victoria D. Schmidt

Contact Antigone Press, LLC though Victoria D. Schmidt at victoriadschmidt.com

Library of Congress Cataloguing-in-Publication Data
LCCN 2016906718

Schmidt, Victoria D.
 Victoria's 95 Secrets
 p.cm.
 ISBN 978-0692711903

PRINTED IN THE UNITED STATES OF AMERICA

ABOUT THE BOOK

"I arrived at her 90th birthday party and waited patiently at the door to enter the home of Victoria Dabrowski Schmidt. This would be my first time meeting her and I did not know this encounter would forever change my life. The door opened and there she was. Victoria with her infectious zesl for life, unspeakable wisdom, grace, beauty, and giving spirit. She immediately embraced me and from that moment on my transformation begun. The opening of the door soon became symbolic of how my life was going to change. She understands her secrets to living a long, meaningful and successful life are to be shared with others. Victoria is living out her purpose to help others. You are not reading her book by chance, it is destined that Victoria's 95 Secrets will metamorphycize your life in positive ways you could never imagine. Get ready for your door to be opened to start living the life you have always wanted! Thank you Victoria for changing the way I see myself and my life and not keeping the secrets to yourself!"

Valerie L. Anderson '81, MBA
Executive Director,
Associate Alumnae of Douglass College,
New Brunswick, NJ 00901

"The moment I met Victoria, I felt renewed. Her sense of being in the world is so bright that you can't help but feel revitalized. She's a pleasure and a joy to engage in conversation and the Secrets in her book, Victoria's 95 Secrets have been a true blessing and of great benefit. Her sage wisdom on the importance of real friendships (especially SECRET #57), the balanced benefits of certain foods (YAY, SALMON in Secret #41) and the powerful purpose of meditation (Secret #26) are just some of the secrets she shares in this timely tome that really helped to change my life and the course of my well-being. You would be hard-pressed to believe that she's 95 years young but her energy, coupled with her dazzling wisdom, proves that her life has been well-lived and well-learned!"

Kevin E. Taylor,
TY Host of "Now What?!
with Kevin E. Taylor," pastor and author.
Newark, New Jersey

I'm very excited about Victoria's 95 Secrets. As a practicing Chiropractor for over 35 years our focus has been to help people in mind body and spirit. Victoria's 95 Secrets is a must read for anyone seeking self improvement not only physically but emotionally as well . Author Victoria D. Schmidt shares her wisdom in an insightful and motivational way . Practical application abounds throughout and you will benefit immediately . These positive and constructive words will resonate with your inner self. Let Victoria's take on life guide and fuel you on your journey ! I endorse and support the valuable concepts put forth in this book. Enjoy !

Dr John G. Murray,
Practicing Chiropractor
Clinton, New Jersey

Victoria's 95 Secrets aren't really secrets at all, rather a reminder (like the first secret) that positive thoughts and surroundings play an integral role in the quality of our lives. Author Victoria D. Schmidt shares her words, experiences and knowledge with the reader in a way that demonstrates easy to follow guidelines for enhancing our lifestyle and prolonging our own lives. This book has many secrets for everyone. For some readers, they may learn from all 95 of them. She has a gift of writing that captivates the reader which made me want to keep reading to learn more. Her desire to help others and to continue her quest for knowledge is evident in this book. She shows that no matter how old one is, there is always something new to learn. Victoria is an amazing woman and a great role model for others. If putting her words to action will help us lead a happy, healthy, long life, may we all incorporate her secrets to feel as young as she does at 95!

Tamra Campanella
Administrative Director, Hunterdon Health
and Wellness Centers, Clinton and
Whitehouse, New Jersey

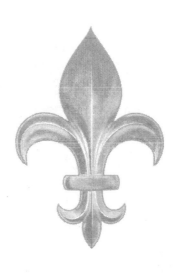

Acknowledgements

My first acknowledgement is not a person. Instead, I credit an incident that inspired me and indicated that a book on my Secrets would attract multitudes of interested readers. After Fox News Television Channel received a copy of my last book, *Move On, Reinvent Yourself, Find Contentment, I Did.* I was asked for a short take on Ways to Live a Long Life for the Fox website. The feature I submitted offered seven Secrets on the subject. After it ran, I had a thousand hits on my website. I went to work on a e-mail newsletter on the subject and now, two years later, I offer my book, Victoria's 95 Secrets.

Since then, there have been scores of individuals to whom I owe gratitude for their support and contributions toward helping me produce my book. I begin with Walter Geslak, a longtime friend who introduced me to Kevin E. Taylor, a pastor, author and TV host. Kevin not only explained the importance of social media for me, he suggested I work with Edward Coutain, I thank Edward for designing, formatting and much of the marketing for Victoria's 95 Secrets as well as for the technical aspects of my social media.

I am honored and deeply grateful to Dr. Howard S. Friedman for his edifying Foreword for my book. Dr. Friedman is Distinguished Professor, University of California, Riverside. Author of Friedman, H. S. & Martin, L. R. The Longevity Project: Surprising Discoveries for Health and Long Life from the Landmark Eight-Decade Study.

Among others I acknowledge are the four who have prepared short reviews that appear in the front of the book: again, Kevin E. Taylor, pastor, author, TV host, Valerie Anderson, Executive Director of the Alumnae Association of my alma mater, Douglass College, Rutgers, The State University of New Jersey, Dr. John A. Murray, Chiropractor and Tamra Campanella, Director of Hunterdon Health and Wellness Centers in Clinton and Whitehouse Station, New Jersey.

I extend my appreciation to Travis Meador for executing the reorganization of my Secrets to manuscript and the book's PPT; editors Elizabeth Cody Kimmel and Kevin Anderson; Artist, Victor Dorobantu, for his descriptive sketches; Nick Romanenko, for the photos of me and Niqui; and Jen Magro, my exercise trainer, who reviewed and supplied information for my exercise Secrets and Emily, her 14-year-old daughter, for tech assistance.

In the back of the book Appendix, I acknowledge by Secret the long list of: experts, researchers, writers, research centers, publications, journals, universities and medical centers whom and that I have credited or quoted.

I express my deepest appreciation to all who have contributed to making *Victoria's 95 Secrets* a source for those who want to live a healthy, happy, sexy, long life

Thank you.

Foreword

It is always a pleasure to see individuals thriving into their 80s, 90s and even beyond. There is a misconception that getting older means illness, pain, and suffering. Quite the contrary, it is those individuals who are destined to die before age 75 who are most likely to be suffering through middle age with heart disease, cancer, depression, diabetes, and more. Author Victoria D. Schmidt is an inspiring example of a long-lived individual who has stayed healthy and fulfilled throughout her life. In her book, she offers her "secrets" on how she continues to live a rewarding, long life.

We do not yet know all the secrets to health, thriving, and long life, but we know a lot, and we know that it is helpful to keep probing and seeking and striving for a successful path you can follow. In my 25 years of work as chief scientific investigator on The Longevity Project (http://www.howardsfriedman.com/longevityproject/), we have discovered a number of healthy pathways, and we have found that each individual needs to seek his or her optimal path. We do know that physical activity is hugely important —staying active through walking or dancing or gardening or just about anything that keeps you up and out of your chair.

We also know that a meaningful life, including dedication to others, can be health-promoting in a variety of ways. And, those who thrive tend to be responsibly prudent, following the things that the mature, wise people in your life have advised. When it comes to food, stress, sleep, and optimism, there is still a lot we do not understand. But we do know that the healthy and thriving life pathways not only often lead to good health and long life, but they also often produce happy times and a sense of well-being. So, stay involved. Perseverance, enthusiasm and dedication go a lot further in unlocking the secrets of good health than we might at first think.

Howard S. Friedman
Distinguished Professor, University of California, Riverside
Author of: Friedman, H. S. & Martin, L. R. The **Longevity Project**: Surprising Discoveries for Health and Long Life from the Landmark Eight-Decade Study.

Introduction

There are two significant reasons why I chose to record my *Long Life Secrets*. The first and most significant is that when I was in my early eighties, my friends (even those in their twenties and thirties) began to ask me about my Secrets for living a happy, healthy, sexy, and long life. On the day I turned 93, I decided to give my friends what they wanted—I would divulge a collection of the Secrets to my vitality in a book. Today as I prepare to celebrate my next birthday, it seems a fitting gift to myself that I finalize this project.

The second reason for sharing these Secrets is my discovery and realization (over the course of my 95 years) of fascinating concepts and theories about specific practices that contribute to living a happy, healthy life. I have investigated them and incorporated those that work for me into my own daily life. I have used these precepts to create the comprehensive Secrets which have previously been available only in an electronic newsletter to a long list of my friends. Now, I have assembled them here in my book.

I can vividly remember being just three or four years old and talking with my young friends about life and how long we might live. In those days, the only clue seemed to be the life-lines in the palms of our hands. To my regret, my lifeline was not as long as my friend Buddy Houser's. But when Buddy died at 17, I began to realize the riddle of longevity was not hidden in the folds of my skin. It was my own to discover and master. It is a lesson I have never forgotten.

I found a wealth of information about various precepts and theories that may contribute to a long life. Much of what I found was presented by respected, knowledgeable experts in the field of longevity—most of whom were in their forties and fifties. I have yet to find a longevity expert who has lived those precepts as I have, and as I continue to do throughout and beyond my 95 years.

It was when I turned ninety-three that I fully realized how fulfilling and exciting a life I had been living, that I decided to share my gift. Hoping that others will be inspired and edified by my experiences, I offer my Secrets, along with my mantra:

*You must **want** to live a long life*
and view living with grace and acceptance.

I do not suggest that you will add years to your life by undertaking all or any of my 95 precepts at once nor even if you practice them regularly. Nor do I include the negatives, those bad habits about which we are constantly reminded to avoid—those that bring on illnesses and shorten our lives.

However, if you do undertake any of my Secrets—*with the proper spirit, in a positive frame of mind and believe that you can*—you may be surprised to find yourself becoming healthier and happier. You can choose to begin with Secret #1, The Power of Positive Thinking, and follow with the six in the Basics Category—without which you cannot live well. Then check the categories in the Table of Contents and/or flip through the Secrets and find those that will help the most during the era you are living now.

Are you a Gen Z? A millennial? A baby boomer? A retiree?

****

Should you seek a mentor? Do you need tech assistance?
How is your balance? Want a fun way to exercise?
Have you lost someone dear to you?
Take on your Secrets and practice them at your own pace, move on and enjoy the years they will add to your life.

Don't ever give up. As you continue to introduce new Secrets into your daily routine, they can become as much a part of your existence as breathing. I have found that as I consciously practice and add new precepts, the earlier ones continue automatically on their own. Though most of my Secrets are purely common sense, we must constantly remind ourselves of the importance of each until they do become a part of our lives.

Make every effort to recognize the full power of positive thinking and rely on the strength of your spirit to guide you. When you put aside the accepted limitations of your age, your gender, your memory and whatever else you think may be standing in your path, you will be on your way to living a healthy, happy, and long life.

Good Luck!

TABLE OF CONTENTS

V. Stress Management

VI. Posture

VII. Fear and Anxieties

VIII. Nutrition - Delectable Healthful Food

XX. Other

XXI. Love Every Year of Your Life

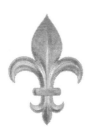

Secret 1
NUMBER
The Power of Positive Thinking

For as long as I can remember, even back when I was a tod-
dler, I always had a sunny outlook on things and rejected the
glass-half-empty view. My sister and her friends, three years
older than I, taunted me occasionally, calling me "Victrola,"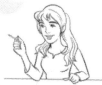
the music player of the times. I chased them up a tall fence, too tall for me to navigate
myself, and thus held captive I would shout, "Victoria is a beautiful name!" In time, I
came to believe it myself.

I have been what some would call an optimist all of my life, and I believe it has
played an important role in how happy and long a life I am living. Friends who have
taken my advice, as the old song goes, to "accentuate the positive, eliminate the negative, and latch on to the affirmative," tell me they have experienced profound changes
in their lives, regardless of their age.

The concept that thought and prayer can heal has been with us for as long as the
human race. Today, it is supported by scientific research and data. Studies have proven
there is a link between heightened stress and certain diseases. The field of psychoneu-
roimmunology, or the study of how emotions and stress affect our immune systems, is
one of medicine's newest branches. Even its name is young, first coined in 1982. Research in this field shows clear evidence of a relationship between thought and health.
In other words, your thoughts can affect your physical well-being. Imagery can make
us ill. It can also help us heal.

So think positive thoughts!
Don't mess with Mr. In-Between

I. The Basic Secrets

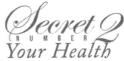

Secret 2
(NUMBER)
Your Health

Aging well is not all in the genes.
Even those with the good ones don't always make it.
If you want to, will it, and do all the right basic things,
or most of them, you will make it! As I have.

The basics of good health are well known, and most of us have heard them time and time again. But in my experience, they are basics for the very reason that they are critical to long life and should be part of one's everyday routine. Start with the most basic building block of longevity: the state of your health. If you haven't had a checkup in over a year, arrange for a complete physical exam with a health provider. Don't worry how long it's been since your last checkup, the doctor will be happy to see you anyway. Don't hesitate to get a second opinion if you are uncertain about your interview or the exam. When you leave or soon after your exam you should know the state of your health and what type of treatment plan you need, if any. Visit your doctor regularly.

Other essential elements of health include diet, self-image, exercise and sleep. You will find them included in my Secrets, along with many Secrets that aren't part of the basics. All contribute dramatically to enjoying and ensuring a long life.

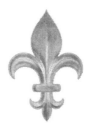

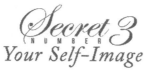

Secret Number 3
Your Self-Image

Develop and/or strengthen your identity, the image you see as your ideal self and the way you hope others will perceive you. Understanding the nature of your self-image—and realizing that you have control over every aspect of it—can put you on the path to longevity. Do you have an identity that feels authentically your own? Or do you relate too closely to the characteristics of someone else: your spouse, a family member, or someone you admire? Discovering and cultivating a self-image that is truly your own can be rewarding and fun. Analyze the qualities you already have and the beliefs you have about yourself.

Which ones are positive or redeeming? Once you know that, you can build on them. Which ones are negative or not serving you well? Having identified them, you can eliminate those qualities or beliefs that contradict your ideal self-image. Consider your sense of style, your appearance, your interests, your relationships, your likes, your dislikes, your opinions, your philosophy—are they an accurate reflection of who you are, or are they conforming to fit the expectations of others? Each one of these elements is a window into your identity, and their blend is what shapes you. Add a touch of vanity if it isn't already there. It won't hurt, and a little vanity may go a long way toward helping.

In making the effort to examine the qualities and beliefs forming your identity, you will learn who you are, decide who you want to be, and project a positive self-image. It will take time, but you may be closer than you think, and the effort is worth it. With a strong, clear, and authentic self-image, you will feel good about yourself, gain greater confidence, and launch your long life.

Secret Number 4
Your Exercise Regimen
Of all the basic, obvious, right things in a long-life plan,
exercise is the most time-exacting,
but working out helps lower the risk of life-threatening diseases.

Your exercise regimen should ultimately include some rigorous workouts. If you are just beginning, try something you do all the time: walking! Just do more of it, at a brisk pace and on a regular schedule. I walk one and a half miles each morning with Niqui, my gentle whippet, exercise a half hour in the late afternoon, and take balance lessons twice a week with a trainer. I love it. As a result, my immune system is strong, my risk of certain conditions and illnesses is reduced, and I'm much less likely to injure myself. Most importantly, my exercise regimen provides constant reinforcement of my view of myself as an independent, strong, and capable person.

There are countless exercise programs of every kind; it only requires a little research to find the best one for you. Whether you want a highly structured class at a well-appointed health club or a simple routine you can do at home, it's out there. You may ask a willing friend to join you. Companionship is healthy and can keep both of you going. If you start a fitness regime during the winter, you'll be in good shape to don your swimsuit in summer—having a payoff in mind can be very motivating.

And of course, make informed decisions about any exercise program and check with your doctor to make sure a regimen is right for you.

Don't let existing physical limitations convince you that an exercise regimen is beyond your capabilities. Whether you have lower-back issues or tricky knees or only one good lung, there is a safe and healthful way for you to exercise. All you have to do is find it.

Among the established programs that are worth investigating are Pilates and Zumba. Both are popular, have millions of enthusiasts, and are taught all over the world.

Once you have launched your exercise regimen,
you will not only be on your path to good health and energy;
you will be on your way to a vigorous, long life.

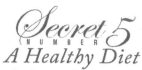

Secret 5
(NUMBER)
A Healthy Diet

What you eat—the foods that make up your diet—is another basic
and obvious element in living a long, healthy life

Our bodies—and the muscles, bones, and organs within them—are designed to work well and maintain themselves, but they need the right kind of fuel to do so. Eating a healthy diet doesn't mean deprivation—it simply involves being aware of the basic needs of your physical system and including foods that provide for those needs. Simply, if you want good health that leads to a long life, eat healthful foods!

This Secret is not about losing or gaining weight. It is perfectly possible to be in good health within a wide range of weights. It offers suggestions on how to attain and maintain good health.

- Cut back or eliminate fatty foods.
- Drink lots of tea.
- Limit (or eliminate if you can) the amount of red meat you eat.
- Indulge in fruits and veggies.
- Substitute olive oil, coconut oil and canola oil for butter.
- Include legumes in your meals. Beans, peas, and lentils help lower cholesterol.
- Fill up on fish. The omega-3 fats in seafood help prevent heart disease.
- Nibble nuts in moderate amounts. Walnuts, almonds, and pistachios provide healthy fats.
- Have a glass of purple grape juice or red wine every day.

These tips provide you with the benefits of fiber, minerals, and antioxidants and help keep your immune system healthy. They lower your cholesterol and help protect you against a wide range of cancers, heart disease, osteoporosis, and diabetes.

Want help with a special problem? Seek out a nutritionist who will design a diet that will take care of your need.

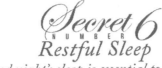

Secret 6
NUMBER 6
Restful Sleep
A good night's sleep is essential to longevity
and a healthy life.

A good night's sleep is a powerful tonic. It can reduce stress and boost your energy, your mood, and your concentration. Plentiful sleep can impact your life in almost every way imaginable, from making you more productive at your daily tasks to providing a sense of well-being. If you are having trouble sleeping, particularly in the summer, you are not alone. According to a survey by Prevention magazine, half of Americans indicate they are so active in the hot-weather months enjoying themselves that they don't have much time to sleep. And a third of our population say they are stressed out most in summer.

Other year-round problems you may want to avoid include having trouble falling off to sleep, experiencing a lighter, fitful sleep and waking up and staying awake for longer periods than you wish.

Here are a few tips on how to ensure you enjoy that good night's sleep:

• The food and snacks you eat during the day affect the quality of your sleep. Avoid breads, pastas, sugary desserts, spices, and saturated fats. Indulge in lean proteins like low-fat cheese, turkey, and fish with dashes of fresh herbs. A cup of herbal tea such as peppermint and chamomile before bedtime is relaxing in itself. Make it a part of your nighttime routine.

• Try some abdominal breathing exercises before hopping into bed.

• Keep your bedroom relatively dark. Draw drapes closed, shut off lamps, and limit the amount of light to a nightlight.

• Keep your bedroom's temperature moderate, neither too hot nor too cold.•
Make sure you have a regimen of exercise, even if it is only a few minutes a day.

• Keep a regular wake-up time and go to sleep on schedule.

Avoid medicines that take a toll on your sleep. Check with your doctor to make sure you have the proper medication.

Relax. Put the pressures and stress of your day behind you. Create a sense of calm with a few minutes of meditation, or read a diverting book, a real book, not an e-book. Do a little sewing, even if it is just stitching a hem or attaching a button, nothing too demanding or creative. These are things I do often.

Actor Robert Duvall, a young eighty-three, goes beyond the need to have a full night's sleep and declares that one of his secrets is taking a "short nap every day." Experts suggest you limit a daily snooze to no more than thirty minutes. On occasion, I'll take two ten-minute pick-up quickies during a day.

Secret Number 7
Repeat the Basics

Repeating the Basic Secrets, along with the Power of Positive Thinking, Secret 1, is essential to living a happy, healthy, long life. The basics are obvious and critical and are covered in some detail in Secrets 2, 3, 4, 5, and 6. I list them again, briefly, here:

Secret 2 is your health. Start with having a complete physical exam and follow with visiting your doctor regularly.

Secret 3 is your self-image. Develop or strengthen your identity and you will feel good about yourself and gain greater self-confidence.

Secret 4 is exercise. If you haven't yet set up an exercise regimen, begin with walking faster and more often. Then explore other programs on the Internet, local health centers, such as the YMCA and YWCA and others. Among the established programs that are worth investigating are Pilates and Zumba. Both are popular, have millions of enthusiasts, and are taught all over the world.

Secret 5 is diet. A few suggestions for a healthy diet include cutting back on fatty food, drinking lots of tea, indulging in fruits and veggies, filling up on fish, and nibbling on nuts.

Secret 6 is sleep. Among the many ways you can enjoy a good night's sleep is to be selective in the foods you eat, do some abdominal breathing exercises before hopping into bed, and put the pressures of the day behind you.

These Secrets should be a part of your everyday experiences. If you have neglected them, then review them and reconsider including them in a regular routine. Not only do they contribute to your living a long life, but you will be surprised how much better you will feel.

II. Happiness

Secret 8

NUMBER

The Benefits of Laughing Out Loud

The human race has one really effective weapon,
and that is laughter. –Mark Twain

Laughter is contagious, infectious, and a powerful way to keep you healthy and add years to your life. It makes you feel great and the feeling stays with you even as the laughter ebbs; the glow of well-being continues. You will view the rest of your day and the world positively and with joy. You will also be more inspired, creative, and productive in your work —or play.

A hearty laugh has benefits that enhance not only your physical health but your mental health and your social life. Scientific research has demonstrated that laughter can have as great an effect on the body as pain medication or antidepressants. But laughs are free, and you can have as many as you want! Try laughing yourself. Start with a smile, continue with a chuckle, and then go onto a guffaw. Keep going even though it may feel a little forced. If you continue you will feel more relaxed, less tense, and more cheerful. Share it with a friend and double the good feeling.

Enjoy the endless benefits of laughter!

Laughter benefits your health by
stimulating several organs, the heart, lungs and muscles
increasing endorphins, the body's natural good feeling chemicals.
relaxing the entire body and relieving pain
protecting the heart against cardiovascular disease
relieving stress and soothing tension

Laughter enhances your social life to
- make upbeat friends
- divert disagreements
- unite family and friends in trying times
- strengthen relationships
- attract positive people

Laughter benefits your mental health by
- helping to cope with problems
- lessening depression
- improving your mood
- relieving stress
- bringing joy and happiness to life

For the most part these benefits are short-term, day-to-day pick-me-ups. However, laughter, repeated regularly—say, at least once every day—may, according to the Mayo Clinic, improve your immune system. Laughter and "positive thoughts release neuropeptides that help fight stress and potentially more serious illnesses."

Laugh. Laugh a lot and often.

Secret 9
(NUMBER)

Ways to Make You Laugh
You can create opportunities that make you laugh.

"He began to laugh, so that his tall, lean body shook, and his long legs couldn't hold him, and he had to lean up against the building, seized with laughter, abundant and unstoppable; and so he leaned in the wild sun, against the stones of the building, with the tears flying from his eyes—full of foolishness, howling, hanging on to the stones, crawling with laughter, clasping his own body as it began to fly apart in the nonsense, the sweetness, the intelligence, the bright happiness falling, like tiny golden flowers, like the sunlight itself, the lilt of Hunt's voice, on this simple afternoon, with a friend, in Pisa." -Mary Oliver, West Wind: Poems and Prose Poems

A great way to enjoy the benefits of laughter that I discuss in Secret 8 is to make sure you have at least one hearty laugh every day. You will be on the path to experiencing one of the most powerful ways to keep you healthy! Your physical and mental health will improve, your social relationships will be enhanced, and you will add years to your life. Laughter is a learnable skill. If you don't have it, you just have to work on it. Here are a few tips to help you have fun and humor in your life.

Prepare yourself to take on the happiness of laughter!
Make a list of your blessings and avoid the negatives
Respond to questions spontaneously
Don't permit yourself to be on the defensive
Be honest and open with your emotions
Create an upbeat mood
Don't take yourself too seriously

Laugh when you are alone	*Laugh with others*
Read the comic strips	Sharing laughter with others is more
Go to a comedy movie or play	powerful than laughing alone!
Get a book of jokes. Read it	Do with others the laughing alones that apply
Join the groups you hear laughing	Make friends who are upbeat and positive
Attend a comedy club	Share jokes and funny incidents from your life
Join a laughter yoga class	Find the humor in the bumps of your own day
Look at yourself in the mirror	

Whether you want to do all or any of the above, I suggest here the best way to have fun and laughter. It is at the top of my list. Adopt a pet or spend more time with yours if you already have one. Mine, a gentle whippet I call Niqui, not only makes me laugh till I cry, she is my devoted companion. Her full title is Dominique, La Princesse de Poitier.

Laugh. Laugh a lot and often.

Secret 10

Smile, Smile Often, and See What Happens
"twice I have lived forever in a smile
—e. e. cummings

Many years ago, when I was in my twenties, I came across a photo feature in a fashion magazine that has had a lasting effect on me. The article was titled "You Can Be More Beautiful, at Times, Than a Fashion Model." It startled me. I never considered myself particularly beautiful. Nor did I have to be as beautiful as a model. I'd settle for pretty or perhaps almost as attractive. There were two photos of the same model—one as she smiled—the other as she frowned. The writer suggested the reader look in the mirror and do the same. I did! I smiled. I looked far better than the frowning model. Since then, I refuse to frown. Whenever I find myself frowning, I smile.

So turn your frown upside down! Smile!

There are far more reasons for smiling than looking beautiful, though feeling beautiful is helpful and uplifting. Studies reveal that there are countless benefits for those who make a practice of smiling regularly. It has been proven that even a fake smile, which can turn into one that is genuine, has amazing effects that make you and those to whom you smile be happy.

Here are some of the reasons that studies have found why you should smile often.

Smiling . . .

. . . can be contagious. I am a constant smiler. I find it doesn't always create a like response, particularly at the gym, where exercisers focus on their routines. Sad! They should be happy as they work out. Walkers and runners are not only great smilers; they eagerly respond with a pleasant greeting . Smiling can:

• put you in a better mood, make you feel more comfortable, and turn your day around.

• make you more approachable and open to potential friends. A smile is inviting and lets people know you are open to talking and socializing.

• help you, if even briefly, to be open to stick to tasks and be more productive in your work.

• cause your system to release endorphins, the same chemicals produced when you run or work out. Smiling is much easier than jogging to achieve a "runner's high."

• strengthen your immune system by helping your body produce more white blood cells to fight diseases.

• make you look younger by giving your face a natural lift.

• help relieve stress by keeping you from holding tension and frowns in your face that keep you stuck in the loop of feeling tired or overwhelmed.

• make you appear confident and successful and can help you remain positive. It is difficult to be negative, worry, or be angry when you turn your frown upside down and smile.

So smile, smile often and see what happens!

III. Lifetime Goals

"Be compassionate. Work for peace in your heart and in the world. Work for peace and I say again never give up. No matter what is happening, no matter what is going on around you. Never give up."

—His Holiness the 14th Dalai Lama

Secret 11
(NUMBER)

Analyzing Goals and Making Decisions

We make the best decisions when we: Go slowly.
Set goals! Have a plan!

From time to time, we all are faced with major changes and must make decisions about which path to take. If you've taken the time to cultivate a strong self-image, your increase in self-confidence will help you make informed, sensible decisions. That doesn't mean some choices won't be hard. But if you know who you are, it's so much easier to know where you want to be going.

Life decisions can create a lot of pressure, but don't be tempted to rush them. They are best approached slowly and with caution. Is your choice in keeping with the goals you have set for yourself? Or will your goals need redefining? Are you offered an opportunity you have hoped for and can't pass up? Don't accept it out of hand—take the time to think through each possibility. Imagine yourself in a year if you choose to move, and imagine yourself in a year if you choose to stay where you are. Can you imagine yourself happy in both scenarios?

Investing the time to analyze your options and situation, review your goals, and establish a plan to accomplish them will make any transition smoother. It will also help you to know that you have made the right choice.

On occasion we are forced to make an instantaneous decision: in traffic, a sudden crisis, an unexpected loss. Before that happens, when you are relaxed and free, try thinking about what life may put in your path. Contemplate and determine what you would do. Remind yourself that there are very few conditions in life in which we cannot be happy. Then, suddenly you are there; you will go into automatic pilot and your reaction will not be at the mercy of panic or fear. I experienced such an incident and avoided a tragic accident.

Be prepared! Good luck!

Page 12

Secret *12*
(N U M B E R
Determining Lifetime Goals

I am a constant goal setter. I have goals of all kinds, from whether to sign up for fencing lessons next week to what big project to take on next. In addition to those, I have two lifetime goals. The first is to live a healthy, happy, rewarding, and long life. The second is to fulfill my mission to help others enjoy the good life as I do. To help you carry out your pursuits with a purpose.

What are goals? Simply, a goal is a desired objective or purpose. There are short-term goals, lifestyle goals, financial goals, but when we are crafting the course of our life, we're guided by long-term goals. *Wikipedia* offers a more comprehensive definition which I shorten here:

> **A goal is a desired result a person envisions,**
> **plans and commits to, to achieve a hoped-for end-point.**

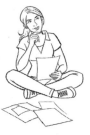

Why set goals? People who are successful in any field of life—business, journalism, politics, the arts, athletics, and many others—know firsthand the value of setting goals. Goals help you focus. You will be able to acquire more data about your field or objective and organize your resources and your time. As you achieve each goal, your increasing confidence and self-esteem help you move on from each short-term goal to your ultimate lifetime goal.

What are some areas in which to consider establishing long-life goals? Career, family, finances, expanding your knowledge in a special field, physical fitness / health, pleasure, volunteerism, to name a few. Select one or two that are important to you and that you feel can sustain you over the long haul. What do you want to achieve in your life? Don't rush. Be sure you set your standards high with lofty but achievable goals. Once you have selected your long-term, lifetime goals, they will act as signposts to keep you on track.

Decision making can be challenging and fun. Enjoy.

Secret № 13
Setting Your Goals

Once you have determined a few lifetime goals, you are ready to move on to the next step of setting short-term, preliminary goals. The length of your short-term goals depends on where you are in your life and how far out your lifetime goal extends ahead of you.

A segment has a series of smaller, short-term goals. It is up to you to create your time-line-schedule as you plan what you hope to achieve. Start with a one-week goal. Then set a one-month goal and then a six-month goal. I've always liked to have goals for the next five years, the next ten years, and every year after that.

When you have set your short-term goals, it's time to get to work. You needn't be rigid and keep precisely to a schedule. You can adjust it depending on your progress. Making a list every day and updating it helps. I change mine often, but the long-term goals keep me focused.

The pundits of goal setting suggest you set SMART goals:
Specific, Measurable, Attainable, Relevant, and Time bound.

The step of setting goals is critical and takes much thought and self-analysis. Is your goal to be an artist, an architect, a singer, a writer, a traveler, a fashion designer, a technology nerd or to improve your health or have a family? Where would you like to be in ten years? Or at the peak of your life? It is never too early, or too late, to set goals.

Here is an apt related story: Douglass College at Rutgers University named a career conference after me. The conference is designed to prepare juniors and seniors to launch their careers. In a conversation with a twenty-year-old student I asked her what her lifetime goal was. She did not hesitate before answering that she wanted to be the Editor-in-Chief of Vogue magazine. She asked me what steps she should take to get there. I told her she had already taken the first step—knowing what she wanted!

Carrying out objectives takes dedication, hard work, and a good work ethic. From time to time I step back and take inventory, to evaluate where I am and whether what I've taken on will get in the way of practicing my Secrets—walking a mile and a half each morning, getting eight hours of sleep every night, having lunch with a friend or colleague three or four times a month, meditating, and all the rest. How do you relax? Taking a walk in the park or spending a summer afternoon on a sunny beach or a weekend sailing? You deserve to enjoy! Always remember, having goals keeps you focused and engaged and adds years to your life. I promise.

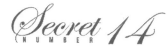

Secret Number *14*
Stay on Course and Reward Yourself

Congratulations! You have now determined your goals and established your timetable for accomplishing them. You are ready to work toward achieving your mission. Write! Write on a yellow pad or type at the top of a page on your computer a clear statement of your lifetime goal, your mission. Intentions are intangible, but when we write them down over and over they become more concrete and immediate. I like to think about my goals, but when I put them down on paper they have special meaning to me:

I want to live a happy, healthy, rewarding long life
and to help others live the "good life," as I do.

Here are some ways to help you stay on course.

Never forget to take some time to indulge yourself by reviewing what you have already accomplished. While it is important to plan ahead, it is also important to be happy in the present moment. Take stock of what you've accomplished; let yourself feel good about you! I take pride in completing each goal. I'm happy to rest on my laurels for a day or two to enjoy the feeling of having set out to do a thing and having done it. But I never linger there too long—there's always the next challenge, moving on to the next level.

I didn't start till I was far along with my current lifetime goal. I needed time to catch up. I now have them neatly arranged and filed in binders for easy reference.

Staying on course ensures you will achieve your lifetime goal(s). When you do, you will have gained confidence and self-esteem and you will find happiness that will add years to your life. You deserve to celebrate and reward yourself with a cruise, a tour, or a lavish party for your friends and those who contributed to your success. You may even choose to treat yourself to the challenge of another lifetime mission.

$\mathcal{Secret}$ 15
Romanticizing Your Goals
Have a quest, a dream

It was in 1965 when I was attending a performance of *The Man of La Mancha* in New York City that I was moved to launch *my* dream.

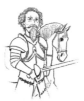

Strive to help others,
no matter how hopeless,
no matter how far!

The theme of the musical expressed through its lyrics and music has become part of me and has defined my life. Of all the songs, *The Quest/The Impossible Dream* has been the most inspirational. It is most powerful for me when I hear it performed by Peter O'Toole. I offer the lyrics here:

The Impossible Dream
Music by Mitch Leigh, lyrics by Joe Darion

To dream the impossible dream
To fight the unbeatable foe
To bear with unbearable sorrow
To run where the brave dare not go

To right the unrightable wrong
To love pure and chaste from afar
To try when your arms are too heavy
To reach the unreachable star

This is my quest
To follow that star
No matter how hopeless
No matter how far

To fight for the right
Without question or pause
To be willing to march into hell
For a heavenly cause

And I know I'll be true
To this glorious quest
That my heart will lie peaceful and calm
When I'm laid to my rest

And the world will be better for this
That one man, scorned and covered with scars
Still strove with his last once of courage
To reach the unreachable star.

I hope this inspires you too as you follow **your** star or you seek inspiration for your dream in other songs that move **you**.

IV. Balance

Secret 16
(NUMBER)

Take Control of Your Sense of Balance

How good is your balance? Strengthening your body brings a sense of independence and will improve your quality of life. Too often adults who are experiencing a loss of balance believe that they cannot regain their earlier muscular strength. You can! The earlier in your life that you start the process, the more likely you will succeed and improve. Nonetheless, even someone in his or her nineties, as I am, can make progress. At ninety-two I began with my trainer, Jen Magro, who is responsible for much of the information in this Secret and has helped me regain confidence and improve my balance.

Though most adults believe that loss of balance is due to aging,
research reveals that it can occur as early as the teen years.

If you sense a need to improve, you can work with an exercise trainer at a gym or local wellness center to learn how to begin. A regular exercise program builds strength, coordination, and endurance. But first, check with your doctor to make sure that your body can handle the exercises.

There are several exercises you can practice yourself to improve, if not completely eliminate, weak balance. You can start with a simple one, the single leg balance. Stand facing a wall with one or both hands against the wall. Lift one foot up in front of you and hold it several inches off the floor while holding a straight posture. When you feel balanced, take one or both hands from the wall and hold the pose for thirty seconds. Repeat the posture with your other leg. Do the exercise five times for each leg, but be careful not to overdo it.

If you still need something more, have your doctor
or an exercise trainer help set up a regimen for you to follow.

Secret 17
Improve Your Balance With Exercise

Balance is a skill like any other, and the more you practice it, the more you improve and become proficient. As years pass we are inclined to slow down, and we tend to limit the everyday energetic activities of living, like taking long walks, playing with our kids (they're grown up), gardening, and other things we used to do regularly. Instead, we choose to relax, sit in the sun, or take a quick dip in the pool rather than doing several laps. Over time, we lose the stimulation that helps maintain the necessary sense of balance.

Are you resigned to losing your balance as years go by and use a cane or a walker?
Or will you begin a regimen now to live
a long, balanced life and walk with a sturdy stride?

There are several factors that contribute to loss of balance:
1. Changes in vision
2. Inner-ear disorders such as vertigo
3. Changes in muscular strength, endurance, and coordination
4. Natural deterioration *(to be blunt, growing old)*

If you have a loss of balance and wish to identify the cause, consult with your doctor, a physical trainer, or an institution like the Mayo Clinic for help.

Mike Ross, an exercise physiologist and author of *The Balance Manual,* has said that doing exercises regularly stimulates the part of the brain that controls balance. The brain learns how to efficiently coordinate all the muscles in your legs and torso that keep you upright and stable.

To achieve any degree of improvement, plan a regular exercise regimen of three to five days a week. Balance exercises put you in a position of *slight instability,* so you must begin by making certain that you are in an environment of *controlled instability.* The exercises are easy and safe. Each requires that you hold on to your support—something sturdy—with one hand, or to have your support nearby to grab onto if necessary.

Two simple ways to practice to improve your balance are

First: Walk heel to toe in a straight line with a cane if you need one.
Second: Stand on one foot and switch to the other while standing near your desk as you talk on the phone, at your kitchen counter preparing a meal, or other places where you can reach a good support.

Here are two exercises from Mike Ross's *The Balance Manual* that you may move on to. First, warm up by holding on to your support, then loosen your grip and gradually remove your fingers until it feels challenging to keep your balance. You may need to keep a couple of fingers on the support, but try to use it as little as possible. Now you're ready for the exercises.

1. The one foot and one toe: Keep one foot flat, and place just the toe of the other foot beside the heel of the flat foot. Reduce your grip, and balance for thirty seconds. Turn around and do it again on the other foot. You will be slightly unstable but your support will help.

2. One foot in front of the other: Hold on to the support and place one foot directly in front of the other. Your sneakers should be touching and form a straight line. Once in position, reduce touching the support as much as possible and hold your balance for thirty seconds. Switch your feet and repeat the position.

If you would like more balance exercises, check *The Balance Manual* and other balance websites on the Internet.

The sooner you begin to strengthen your body and cultivate control of your balance, the sooner you will gain a sense of independence, improve your quality of life, and increase the number of happy years you will live.

V. Stress Management

Secret *NUMBER* 18

Dealing With Stress and Boredom

*Social media is universally intriguing
and can relieve you of boredom and stress.*

Stress and boredom should be avoided like the plague (I do just that) since they contribute to poor health, make you vulnerable to depression, and keep you from enjoying life. I reference Rex Huppke, the self-proclaimed "America's most beloved workplace columnist," who is "easily distracted and routinely succumbs to the siren song of social media."

Huppke calls upon a study by Gloria Mark, a professor at the University of California, Irvine, on how the use of technology can affect people. Her findings indicate that when used properly, social media can rescue you from the potentially debilitating issues of boredom and stress.

When you are focused and working hard, you risk becoming stressed out, and when you lack an all-encompassing interest, you risk becoming bored. Mark's study reveals that taking a brief break by sending an e-mail or going on Facebook may "slowly ease you into a more engaging and productive state." You can learn more about Gloria Mark's study at www.ics.uci.edu/-gmark/.

Imagine! Try it! You may like it and lengthen your life.

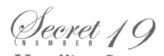

Secret Number 19

Handling Stress
Thoughtful managing of stress will help lengthen your life.

A simple stress management plan of abdominal breathing, relaxation postures, and meditation will help you relax and refresh your spirit, body, and mind. It is wise, if you are not already there, that you begin with practicing abdominal breathing, which is one way to practice conscious breathing.

The poet John Keats refers to breathing in his narrative poem Endymion:

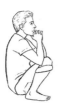

"A thing of beauty is a joy forever;
Its loveliness increases; it will never
Pass into nothingness; but still will keep
A bower quiet for us, and a sleep
Full of sweet dreams, and health, and quiet breathing."

It helps to understand how your body relaxes and reacts when you take deep, conscious breaths. The act of breathing is the only bodily function that is both voluntary and involuntary. The rapid shallow breaths of chest breathing (involuntary) do not bring in large amounts of oxygen to our blood, and thus fewer nutrients are delivered to our body tissue. Abdominal breathing (voluntary), influences the nervous system, which regulates body functions we ordinarily can't control: blood pressure, heart rate, circulation, digestion, and others. Most importantly, abdominal breathing will relax you and you will experience an overall sense of well-being because breathing with awareness lessens and may even eliminate tension and stress.

Always, Breath Mindfully.

Secret Number 20
Understanding the Symptoms of Stress

The symptoms of stress manifest themselves in several ways, and there are few of us—if any—who don't have them. The dictionary definition of stress is "the state of extreme difficulty, pressure and strain." The elements of the condition include

Physical effects: feelings of tension and nervousness, stomach pains and related disorders, diarrhea and constipation, headaches, heart palpitations, and sleeping problems.

Emotional effects: sudden mood swings, diminished interest in sex, overindulgence in eating, drinking, spending or gambling, inability to control events you used to be able to handle, and the desire to escape responsibilities.

Mental effects: confusion, inability to concentrate, momentary loss of memory, and difficulty in expressing yourself.

You may experience these symptoms individually or all at once, and they may vary in intensity. However, even one or two for a short period can take a toll on your life and longevity. Nancy Ferrari, managing editor of Harvard Medical Publications, writes: "Untreated symptoms of stress can lead to chronic physical illnesses that are more difficult to treat than the stress itself."

Not to worry. There are many ways to help stress melt away. However, if you find your symptoms are getting out of hand, consult your doctor for professional help.

Secret Number 21

What Type of Breather Are You?
Determine whether you are a chest or abdominal breather.

Learning what type of breather you are will help put you on the path to eliminating stress. Developing a regimen for abdominal breathing is a must. Abdominal breathing is the proper way to inhale enough oxygen into your blood to support your physiological needs and empower your organs, muscles and limbs. Try this simple test to determine whether you are a chest breather or an abdominal breather.

Start by placing your right hand on your chest, your left on your abdomen. Then take a deep breath, slowly inhaling through your mouth or nose, whichever is natural for you. If your right hand moved more than your left and your shoulders went up, you are a chest breather.

If your left hand rises more than your right, your rib cage expands and most of the movement is in your belly area, then, you already are on your way—you are an abdominal breather. You have pushed your belly out and spurred the flow of oxygen, a major contribution to handling stress.

Don't worry if you are a chest breather.
You can easily learn to be a conscious abdominal breather.

Secret Number 22

Abdominal Breathing Exercises

Abdominal breathing exercises are essential for eliminating stress. Yoga is a form of exercise in which all physical movements begin with the breath. Learning the procedures can be challenging at first but with patience and practice your movements can become fluid and rhythmic.

Allow five to ten minutes for each of the following steps and perform them at least once a day. Even better, do them twice daily:

Step 1: Relax. Sit comfortably on the floor in a cross-legged position or in a straight-backed chair as upright as possible. Rest your hands in your lap, palms up or down.

Step 2: Your eyes may be open or closed. If open, concentrate on an object—a candle, flower, doorknob, lamp—something that doesn't move so you develop a sense of focus. If you close your eyes, focus on the "third eye center," the point between the eyebrows. Quiet your mind and rid yourself of pressing issues and concerns. Focus on the moment and be conscious of your breathing.

Step 3: Begin by drawing in your breath deeply and evenly through both nostrils. Your diaphragm will pull air into the bottom of your lungs and inflate your abdomen. Pause a moment at the top of the inhale.

Step 4: Now, exhale evenly, again through both nostrils. Feel your abdomen pull in, then pause at the end of the exhale. Your breaths should be even in length, about four counts for the exhale until you are proficient with the lengths. Then you may lengthen the exhales.

Step 5: The exercise is complete. Relax. Repeat the steps five times.

Secret 23
Enjoy the Benefits of Abdominal Breathing

Abdominal breathing techniques will calm your mind and body and help eliminate stress. Once you have practiced the exercises in Secret 22 several times and conquered the basic principles, you may add a bit of levity to enjoy your sessions even more. Just say a few words or phrases to yourself that express the emotions you feel as you inhale and exhale. Try words like contentment, relaxation, peace, happiness, beauty, sunset, or any positive word or thought for inhaling. For exhaling, whisper words like stress, anxiety, pain, grrrr, or any negative words. You'll have fun, manage your stress, and add years to your life.

Carolyn Geiger, a qualified yoga instructor at the Hunterdon Health and Wellness Center in Whitehouse Station, New Jersey, has reviewed the yoga procedures in chapter 7 of my book *Move On: Reinvent Yourself, Find Contentment, I Did!*, in which I include a few of hers. All are the basis of my yoga instructions. Carolyn recommends working with a qualified yoga instructor, if not regularly, at least to get you started on your abdominal breathing regimen.

Secret 24

The Practice of Relaxation Postures

Relaxation postures are designed to keep you in touch with your entire body. On the other hand, conscious abdominal breathing keeps you in touch with your bodily functions. Postures are not physical exercises, though you must exert yourself to move into them. They are stances to which you maneuver to make your body supple and flexible and to induce relaxation. The movements unify your body with your mind, your breath, and your nervous system.

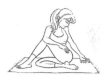

Most postures are derived from the ancient traditions of yoga, and there are countless poses. All take patience and perseverance to perform. The results are worth the effort, for they improve several areas of your health, help control stress, and prepare you for the practice of meditation.

Postures fall into several categories, which include warm up, seated, inversions, forward bends, standing, twist, balance, and Savasana.

You can find additional information on yoga practices in chapter 7 of my book *Move On: Reinvent Yourself, Find Contentment, I Did!* and on the Internet—or sign up for instructions with a qualified yoga instructor at your community gym, wellness center, or yoga studio.

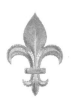

Secret Number 25

Prepare for Relaxation Postures

Prepare correctly, when you choose to carry out
your "long life" relaxation postures at home, on your own.

There are dozens of relaxation postures to choose from when you practice at home (or at a studio). Often, you will find that the name describes the pose. The most common are the Triangle, the Butterfly Mudra, Cat, Upward Facing Dog, Downward Facing Dog, the Plough, the Tree, and the Warrior. The most basic and restorative poses include Child's Pose, Sun Salutation, and Corpse Pose (or Savasana).

Here are items to consider as you prepare for do-it-yourself postures at home using written instructions to guide you:

1. Select a clean, uncluttered, quiet room or a corner that is filled with fresh air from a slightly opened window. Avoid distractions from a television or phone.

2. Wear loosely fitting, comfortable, breathable clothing and perform in bare feet.

3. Place a yoga mat or several large, cushy terry cloth towels on the floor.

4. Do not eat a large meal for at least two hours before your session.

5. Read and reread the instructions before you start each posture. Since it is difficult to read as you practice, consider taping them and listening as you work.

6. You may create a mood in your practice area by playing DVDs of soothing sounds like water rushing in a stream, wind rustling through leaves, a favorite melody—anything to help you relax.

It's wise to first learn the basics with an instructor, then continue on your own. Regardless, check with your doctor first to make sure your body is in sound physical condition to safely handle the routines.

Secret 26

Meditation Clears Your Brain

Meditating trains your mind to eliminate stress

The practice of meditating goes beyond simply lowering stress. It is the act of training and emptying your mind by focusing on one sound, one word, one object, or one thought to free it of all other distractions. You will become more conscious of yourself by slowing down the sense of time passing—something that is critical in today's technological and rapidly changing world. You will be able to better control your moods and thoughts before they overwhelm you and drag your psyche into desperation.

Meditation has been scientifically proven to improve your health. The practice can lower blood pressure and heart and pulse rates, relieve insomnia, and lower the body's core temperature, all of which tend to extend your life. Your mind will be more alert, your reactions quicker, and your understanding greater.

Secret 27

Create Your Space for Meditation

Where and when you choose to meditate is as critical to achieving the relaxation you seek as the meditation itself. If you can, establish a meditation area. The elements to consider include the size, the location, and the objects with which you surround yourself. The goal is to create an ambience that will help you relax and separate you from your daily pressing concerns and the daunting tasks you face.

The area can be any size—a tiny corner in your bedroom, a nook in the kitchen, even a closet or a whole room if you have the space. But it should be private and quiet with no distractions and your very own retreat.

The objects you select for your meditation area should be intimate and memorable, relate to tranquility, and have special meaning within themselves or for you. You don't need to have them all as I suggest below, but choose as many as you wish to make you feel comfortable, serene and prepared to meditate.

1. Start with a small table or low shelf on which you place a colorful scarf directly or in a tray or on a mat. You may enjoy looking for and finding a puja cloth to use—a two-sided, printed sink runner that is used during a Hindu ritual.

2. In the center of your cloth, place a candle in a votive holder (to avoid a fire) and away from flammable materials. You may select your candle by color, since color has symbolic significance: blue for healing negative emotions; violet or indigo for spirituality; green for your body and mind; orange for energy; and yellow for joy and happiness.

3. Surround your candle with familiar objects: flowers, a favorite book, a typed quotation, a photograph, a small painting, a statue or a figurine, a small water fountain—whatever is soothing and helps you relax.

Your meditation area need not be large or elaborate. It should be a place of peace and one in which you are comfortable.

It is up to you to create your own unique meditation area.

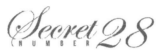

Secret 28

Add a Fragrance to Your Meditation Area

Surrounding yourself with a fragrance when you meditate is soothing and helps you keep in touch with your emotions. You may burn incense or fill your space with the fresh scent of flowers, herbs, fruit or mint that will ensure an ambience of serenity. During the 1930s Dr. Edward Bach, an English physician, developed flower essences to help the healing process. Select a favorite for your place of meditation from among these essences:

- *Arnica treats your trauma.*
- *Sage contributes to your wisdom.*
- *Lavender calms you.*
- *Impatiens helps you accept.*
- *Peppermint and spearmint cool and invigorate you.*
- *Lemongrass lifts your spirits.*
- *Sandalwood soothes your mind.*

All you need to reap the benefits of the scent you choose are a few drops of the oil in a cup of very hot water, which will diffuse and fill your meditation area with a steaming, soothing fragrance.

Now you are ready to melt away your stress!

Secret 29
Enjoy a Sense of Peace by Meditating

With an area prepared, you are ready to begin the practice of meditation itself.

Step 1: In a comfortable chair, or a firm cushion on the floor, sit poised and alert with your back erect and relaxed but not rigid. Avoid a reclining position on a sofa or bed so you aren't tempted to fall asleep. You may have a pillow for your back to make you more comfortable and a throw handy if you get a chill.

Step 2: Select a specific time of day (early morning is best for many) and decide the length of time for each session when there will be no distractions. Plan your session for the same time every day.

Step 3: Close your eyes or fix your gaze on an object or in space several feet away.

Step 4: Select a word, phrase, or thought to focus on, such as love, beauty, peace, home, or springtime in Paris—whatever has a serene meaning for you. Dr. Herbert Benson, a professor at Harvard Medical Institute and founding president of Benson-Henry Institute for Mind Body Medicine at Massachusetts General Hospital, suggests that if you select a mantra that focuses on a spiritual word, you will "achieve deep healing changes within your body and mind." Many meditators use the word om (rhymes with home), which is considered a sacred sound in the Buddhist and Hindu traditions. Another suggestion is shanti, which means "peace." Some find it easier to focus on breathing by thinking "in" on the inhale and "out" on the exhale.

Step 5: Consciously relax every part of your body from the top of your head to your toes. Start with your forehead as you breathe in. Begin to let go of the tension in your body and the stress in your mind as you breathe out. Slowly—always breathing gently—shift your awareness to your eyes, then your nose, mouth, chin, neck, shoulders, and so on, all the way down to your toes. Never stop focusing on the object or mantra you've chosen as your scanning your body. Return your thoughts slowly up your body to the top of your head. Repeat—down and back up.

Step 6: Breathe naturally, maintaining a passive attitude and ignore or set aside any intrusive sounds or thoughts. The object of meditation is not to do it perfectly—it is to notice when thoughts or physical distractions arise and send them away like little clouds, returning to the empty blue sky of silence.

Step 7: When you begin, work with a short period of time, perhaps five minutes. As you become more experienced, increase your time to ten or fifteen minutes.

You may open your eyes to check the time but do not set the alarm. When you have finished your session, you may open your eyes, wait a minute or two before you stand. Rocking back and forth on your feet for a moment will help you get going and move on to the business of your day.

> *If at first you don't sense the peace you expect,*
> *don't give up. It may take two or three sessions*
> *to ensure deep restfulness and serenity.*
> *Just make sure you always maintain a positive attitude.*
> *Enjoy the experience.*

Secret 30
Stress Is Not Always Bad

Working hard and overlong hours, or even into the night, can create stress. I do this often, and with passion. But is stress always a bad thing? Here is what Howard S. Friedman, Distinguished Professor of Psychology at the University of California, relates in his book, The Longevity Project:

> *Those who work the hardest, live the longest.*
> *The responsible and the resourceful achievers thrive in every way,*
> *especially if they are dedicated to people and things beyond themselves.*

There are two kinds of self-induced stress. There is the physical stress that comes from exercising—working out to stretch (stress) our muscles to make them stronger—which is a good thing. Then, there is work stress, as described above, which can strengthen our brain function and increase our capacity to accomplish what we set out to do—another good thing. Both are critical to the development of our bodies and minds.

Controlled stress can motivate you, charge you, and energize you to be more productive by creating a sense of urgency to achieve your goals. How much we should evoke is difficult to determine and different for everyone. Over the years the view of stress has evolved from what my husband Ralph, an accomplished, natural athlete, would say, "No pain, no gain." Today, Jen, my physical trainer is cautious. She suggests avoiding pain and stopping an exercise when it becomes uncomfortable and too stressful.

Though researches have yet to determine finite degrees of controlled stress there are a few guidelines that help manage how far to proceed, either with physical exercise or in your work:

- Press yourself gradually, in moderation, just beyond where you were before. Try to work more efficiently each time you move forward.

- Take time out to give your body and mind time to rest, catch up, and recuperate.

- Maintain your health with a proper diet, a good night's sleep, and a strong sense of purpose.

- Listen to music that you like.

Stress can be a wake-up call to encourage you to reassess where you are in your life. It may be a reminder to take a strategic break and reexamine your goals. You may be bored and need a more challenging goal. Or perhaps you should have a more positive approach to your current project(s) to reaffirm that you are on the right path.

Always remember, stress is not always a bad thing.
It is natural and helpful.
You may need only to take time out and rest.

VI. Posture

Secret 31

The Benefits of Maintaining Proper Posture

Standing, sitting, and walking tall combine to stretch not just your physical frame but your life span. The benefits of maintaining good. posture go beyond just looking positive and poised:

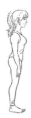

- Your body will function properly.
- You will avoid chronic back, neck, and shoulder pain.
- Your blood will circulate more easily, which can help prevent deterioration of your vertebrae and improve the strength of your muscles and joints.
- You will be able to eliminate stress and elevate your self-esteem.

What constitutes good postures that contribute to a long, healthy life? Here are some basic dos and don'ts:

- Make sure you wear shoes that provide the best support.
- If you wear heels, limit the length of time you wear them.

First check how you stand. It does not mean keeping your spine totally straight:

- Stand with your back to a wall, with your fanny and shoulder blades touching the wall.
- Move your feet forward so your heels are six inches from the wall.
- Place the back of your head—as close as you comfortably can—against the wall.
- Maintain the natural arch of your lower back, a few inches from the wall.
- Tighten your tummy muscles and keep the upright position.
- Bend your knees slightly.
- Keep the back of your arms and shoulders as close to the wall as you can, fingers at your hips.

You should have achieved good standing posture
(If you feel any of the above are uncomfortable or if you have
pain, relax. Or consult a trainer or other professional.)

Next, check your sitting posture:

- Sit on a chair or a bench so your knees are slightly lower than your hips.
- Have your feet flat on the floor and relax your back.
- Keep your head straight ahead, neither up or down.
- Place your shoulders slightly back.

You should have achieved a good sitting posture. Now, check your walking posture:

- Have your chin parallel with the ground.
- Your heel should hit the ground first; then roll onto your toe.
- Hold your tummy and fanny in line with the rest of your body.

You should have achieved a proper walking posture.

A general suggestion for all postures: keep your shoulders firm and slightly back, abs and gluts (fanny) drawn in, and legs securely in place. Now you are prepared to practice the ways to improve your posture.

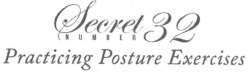

Practicing Posture Exercises

*Practicing good posture can bring about happiness,
confidence, and a positive mood.*

Posture is more than how you stand. It is also about how you sit, walk, and move. The first step in improving your posture is to determine why you want good posture.

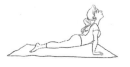

Knowing why will help you achieve your goal.

Do you want to improve your image? Do you want to feel better about your body? Do you want others to have a better perception of you? Do you want to be happy, confident, positive, and poised? Or do you want them all?

Here are some dos and don'ts to help you enjoy the benefits of good posture:

• Keep constantly aware of your posture. Try to develop ways that remind you to maintain good posture. Place a red Post-it note on your computer, your mirror, refrigerator, calendar, exit door, or wherever you feel will help you most.

• Have a good chair and back cushion that are firm and dense.

• Avoid bad habits like sitting on the edge or middle of your chair or working with a dim light (both cause you to slouch and hunch) or lying down reading or watching television. They encourage bad posture. Sit far back in your chair against your cushion.

• Avoid lifting or carrying heavy items. The practice will eventually lead to hunching your shoulders and back. If you must, use a trolley or roller bag.

• Stand up and stretch at least twice every hour, especially if you sit for most of your work day.

• Periodically indulge in a neck, shoulder, and back massage to loosen your joints and help you ease into the good posture position.

• Remember to keep your chin parallel to the ground when you walk. Pay attention to your footfall, starting with your heel first, then rolling onto your toe. Keep your tummy and fanny in line with the rest of your body.

Having an exercise regimen that strengthens your back—
like Pilates, yoga, or sit-ups—contributes largely to achieving good posture.
Keeping your weight down can do wonders.

VII. Fear and Anxieties

Secret 33

Understanding Fears and Anxieties

You can manage the mild
but call on professionals for the chronic and traumatic.

There are times in each of our lives when we find ourselves feeling fear or anxiety. The experience can be as simple as having to take an exam or something more frightening and unpredictable like anticipating a terrorist attack, a reality in today's world.

What is fear? What is anxiety?

Dictionaries define fear as having misgivings of pain about an impending apprehension or evil. Anxiety is concern for a future event that disturbs the mind and keeps it in a painful uneasiness. Dr. Christa McIntyre-Rodriguez, head of the undergraduate neuroscience program at the University of Texas, defines them more simply: "While fear is an immediate response, anxiety is the anticipation of danger."

What are typical fears and anxieties?

Here are just a few: anticipating a job interview, the possibility of being fired, losing a job or a client, pitching a potential client, meeting future in-laws, getting married, having a baby, driving on an icy road, being told you have an incurable disease, competing in a sport or intellectual contest, flying even a short distance—the list is endless. Anxiety exists by creating more anxiety.

The best and easiest way to deal with fear and anxiety
is to take a walk in nature.

According to the Center for Spirituality and Healing, studies in the field of nature-based therapies indicate that being in nature reduces fear and anxiety and increases pleasant feelings. You will experience calm, hope, beauty, happiness, and a greater sense of well-being. Immersing yourself in nature will not only make you feel invigorated; it lowers the heart rate, muscle tension, blood pressure, and stress hormones.

Enjoy the benefits of nature by walking or a running, alone or with a friend, in a park, in the woods or along a nature trail. Not only will you feel physically better, your mood will be uplifted and you will view the world with joy.

There are many substantive ways to conquer mild fears and anxieties. However, if you (or others you know) have experienced trauma or suffer intense chronic fears or anxieties, it's best to seek professional help.

Secret 34

Handling the Lesser Fears and Anxieties

You can handle the less severe anxieties and fears on your own.

"Taking a new step, uttering a new word,
is what people fear the most." —Fyodor M. Dostoyevsky

A good place to start to handle your fears and anxieties and ensure a healthy life is to understand their meanings. I define them at length and then condense them in Secret 33: Fear is an immediate response. Anxiety is the anticipation of danger.

(Keep in mind that the suggestions included here are not for those who suffer trauma or intense chronic fears or anxieties. Those should seek professional help.)

There are steps you can take to prepare yourself as you face both fears and anxieties that will extend the span of your life. Most importantly, build social relationships. Seek support from friends and family who will help you assess realistically what threatens you. Discussing your emotions with those with whom you are close gives you a sense of calm, belonging, and confidence. They will benefit as much as you.

Avoid being in denial. Don't sidestep your negative feelings—accept them. Observe them and understand how they affect your body and psyche. A positive way to face denial is to practice the techniques of yoga and meditation as I discuss in other Secrets. Sit quietly, be in the present, recognize fears and anxieties, but don't try to change them or discard them.

Take time out to evaluate why you are fearful or anxious. Learn what you have control over rather than focusing on what you are not able to handle. Don't permit the negative to drive you. Develop a sense of control and concentrate on your positive attributes. Consider the Serenity Prayer of American theologian Reinhold Niebuhr:

"God, grant me the serenity to accept the things I cannot change,
Courage to change the things I can,
And wisdom to know the difference."

Secret Number 35

Processing Fears and Anxieties

How you can face fear or anxiety.
Consider the statement President Franklin Roosevelt in 1932:
"The only thing to fear is fear itself."

Fear is an immediate response. A few years later when I was a college senior and the Japanese bombed Pearl Harbor, my reaction and those of my classmates were instantaneous. We were stunned and feared the disasters of war. However, our country responded in the most meaningful manner. We found a sense of purpose and unified to reestablish a sense of security. The unity was palpable. Of course we won! I have never experienced such a coming together in my life since.

What do you fear? Everyone has fears. We can be afraid of flying, the dark, heights, snakes, spiders, falling, being attacked on a deserted street, and an infinite number of other things. I have a fear of heights, and something that is more like disgust—I abhor stink bugs, their smell and their shape. Ugh!

We do have the means to process certain fears. For example, you are awakened in the middle of the night by a crashing noise. An intruder? Lights on reveal your dog knocked over the broom you forgot to put back in the closet. You are relieved and laugh. According to Dr. Christa McIntyre-Rodriguez head of the neuroscience program at the University of Texas, a part of your brain helps you through the fear process. For other, more lasting fears like bad news, losing a job, rejection by a friend, or the specter of illness, work in the short term to distract yourself from the emotion when it spikes. Acknowledge the fear, understand it, accept it. Think positively with words like calm, serenity, hope, beauty, happiness. Treat yourself to something indulgent—a gourmet dinner at your favorite restaurant, a massage, a movie, a play, a concert—whatever will distract you. Treat yourself as you would a dear friend in the same spot. You deserve it!

Anxiety is the anticipation of danger. Having an upcoming job interview, an exam, or a speech to deliver before a large audience, all cause anxiety because we tend to worry about them long before the moment is upon us. The fear and the stress may all be in our imagination, but the physical response of the body is the same. Dr. Alan Podawitz, chairman of psychiatry and behavioral health at the University of North Texas Health Science Center, says that prolonged anxiety can lead to physical problems like high blood pressure, lack of appetite and being unable to fall asleep.

Nonetheless, he and other experts indicate that anxiety is part of normal human emotions. It's helpful to ask ourselves, "At the end of the day, will my worrying about this now have any effect on the outcome?" Chances are the answer is no. Dr. Podawitz says the best way to avoid the stress of anxiety is to prepare for it. What is the worst that can happen? It won't. If you are going for a job interview, will the interviewer beat you up? Of course not. You will be asked about your experience, so you should be ready and prepare your response. Your heart rate will slow and your muscles will relax. "It is what the military do before an encounter," Podawitz says. "Yoga and meditation will also help."

Always remember, you can count on nature
to dispel your fears and anxieties.
Take a walk or run, alone or with a friend,
in a park, the woods, or a nature trail.
You will feel better physically, your mood will be uplifted,
and you will view the world with joy.

VII. Nutrition:
Delectable Healthful Foods

Secret 36

The Pleasures and Benefits of Chocolate

Don't eat just any chocolate—,
indulge in the one that's most healthful.

Sometimes it seems like there is an unending stream of new findings about all the things that may be bad for our health. What a pleasant change to have chocolate added to the list of things that can be good for us. It's important to read past the headline, however. Most health benefits are ascribed to organic dark chocolate with 70 percent or higher cocoa content. Most dark chocolates contain some sugar but usually in small amounts. The darker the chocolate, the less the sugar.

Marie Antoinette suggested the French populous eat cake. She should have offered chocolate instead. She may have lived a longer life.

There are many benefits in chocolate;
the most delightful is its undeniably marvelous taste.

When I reached the age of ninety, I began to wonder what it was that might contribute to my longevity. Yes, I do most all the right things mentioned in Secret 2. However, as I began my research and learned about chocolate, this delectable candy may be among my most important Secrets—I'm an unrepentant chocoholic!

Cardiologist and Everyday Health columnist T. Jared Bunch, MD, provides an expert opinion. He recommends, "Dark chocolate should be part of a life plan that includes exercise, eating healthy foods that are largely plant-based, getting adequate sleep, stress reduction and maintenance of weight."

Here are seven of the benefits of dark chocolate
noted in an Everyday Health report.

• Chocolate of the darkest kind is very nutritious. Quality dark chocolate contains adequate amounts of soluble fiber and is rich in minerals: iron, magnesium, copper, manganese, and others.

- Dark chocolate is a powerful source of antioxidants.
- Dark chocolate may improve blood flow in the arteries and lower blood pressure.
- Dark chocolate raises HDL (high, good, density cholesterol) and protects LDL (bad) against oxidation. It can even improve risk factors for heart disease and diabetes.
- Dark chocolate may lower the risk of cardiovascular disease.
- Dark chocolate may protect your skin against the sun.
- Dark chocolate may improve your brain function.

Though dark chocolate boasts these benefits and more, don't overindulge. Dark chocolate is loaded with calories. Enjoy one or two chunks a day and make sure you select the best you can find.

For in-depth details on the benefits of dark chocolate visit
www.everydayhealth.com.

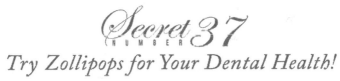

Secret 37
NUMBER

Try Zollipops for Your Dental Health!

A nine-year-old Michigan girl named Alina Morse has come up with a product that keeps your breath fresh and balances your mouth's pH, a measure of how acidic the mouth is after a meal. Zollipops are lollipops sweetened with the sugar substitutes erythritol, xylitol and stevia.

Alina is an old hand at inventing and keeps a notebook full of new ideas. She began when she was three but it took her six years to come up with a winner. (Better than most inventors!) One day, when she was in the bank with her father, she refused the lollipop the teller offered her. Her dad had told her that sugar is not good for teeth. The bright youngster knew that "your mouth is very acidic and your enamel is soft after you eat, so if you brush right after, you hurt the enamel."

She is a typical fourth grader but is inquisitive and asks loads of questions about everything she encounters. On her way home from the bank, she told her father she wanted to make a "healthy sucker that's good for your mouth."

Her father, Tom Morse, a product manufacturer consultant, and her mother, Suzanne, collaborated with Alina and invested $7,500 to make Alina's dream a reality. They conferred with dentists and hygienists.

They spent hours testing ingredients and designing packaging until they had the product they sought: Zollipops, which sell for six dollars a bag of fifteen and are available on amazon.com and elsewhere, had sales of almost $75,000 in their first year.

Want something sweet to eat that sweetens your breath
and keeps your mouth healthy?
Try Zollipops!

Secret 38
A New Spin on Potatoes
Whites are now good for you!

I have always relished mashed white potatoes doused with rich gravy along with two veggies and a portion of chicken or fish for my evening meal. But I felt guilty about the potatoes. No more! White potatoes are okay, but give up most of the gravy.

White potatoes have benefits—different from but equal to sweet potatoes.

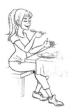

We have been told to avoid white potatoes, mainly because in many popular forms, such as French fries or potato chips, they are highly processed and thus contribute to obesity and the risk of diabetes.

Early this year, the prestigious Institute of Medicine announced that people are not getting enough of the starchy nutrients that are abundant in potatoes. Another government agency, the Women, Infants, and Children's Program, permits the use of certain vegetables, including white potatoes, without added sugars, fats, or oils.

Sweet potatoes have been considered better than whites, since they are usually eaten whole and are a good source of several vitamins. But when fried, they too are usually best avoided.

Scientifically, white and sweet potatoes have complementary benefits and differences. Sweet potatoes are rich in nutrients and have more fiber and vitamin A and a lower glycemic index than whites. White potatoes are higher in essential mineral like iron, potassium and magnesium. *So indulge in sweet or white but avoid the processed foods.*

Secret NUMBER 39
The Vigor of Vitamins
Start with a healthy diet then add the vitamins.

My doctor tells me he considers the vitamins I take a major contribution to my longevity. I began taking vitamins early on, but I never relied on them for all the nutrients I needed—I always took them to complement a healthy diet. I began taking vitamins when my husband, a chemical engineer, and I were first married and he launched his pharmaceutical career. We started with B vitamins, which he was producing at the time. Over the years, with recommendations from our doctors, we added more.

The vitamins and supplements we took and those I take now include

B_{12}	D_3	DHEA	Milk thistle
B complex	Glucosamine/chondroitin		Omega-3
Calcium	Lecithin		Selenium
Coenzyme Q-10	Magnesium		Zinc

The benefits of these vitamins and supplements range from supporting heart and blood-vessel functions, teeth, bone and immune health, and cellular energy production in the body to promoting sugar metabolism, joint health, nerve and heart health, and more. Recently, my optometrist suggested I add Lutein, which supports eye health. I did.

Sound complicated? Many people think so. But you can try a simpler yet reliable way to benefit from vitamins recommended by the Harvard T. H. Chan School of Public Health. Build on a foundation, of course, of a healthy diet that is rich in fruits, vegetables, whole grains, nuts, and healthy oils and low in red meat and unhealthy fats. Then take one multivitamin every day. Add one each of vitamin D and E and a low dose of folic acid, but go easy on that one. The Chan School suggests avoiding "mega-dose" vitamins and "super" supplements and that you check with your doctor or a qualified health provider for a proper vitamin regimen.

Though a schedule of taking vitamins every day
seems like a time consuming project, it's not.
Developing one gradually over a period of time
becomes a subconscious habit and can add years to your life.

Secret 40
Herbs and Spices
Offer More Than Exciting Flavors

Most of us sprinkle our food with salt and pepper to taste and add salt to bring out the flavor of our veggies, meat, and fish as we cook. I also like to throw in a dash of a particular herb or spice from time to time when it is on the list of ingredients of a recipe I'm preparing. Unless we are great or even passable chefs, we are limited to those we use regularly and perhaps one or two more that we have grown up with. Few of us are aware that besides adding exciting flavors to dishes, there are countless numbers of herbs and spices that abound with health benefits. They have antibacterial and antiviral properties, are high in B vitamins and trace minerals, most contain more antioxidants than vegetables and fruits, and some add years to our lives.

Here is a short list of those most often used, the dishes to which to add them, along with some of their benefits:

Basil: add to eggs, vegetables. soups, meats, salads; has anti-inflammatory and antiviral properties and lessens digestive disorders.

Cayenne: add in small amounts to almost any dish, meat, vegetable, or sauce; helps improve absorption of other nutrients and increases circulation.

Cinnamon: for sweet, savory, and chili dishes; provides manganese, iron, and calcium; has high antioxidant value; and can prolong the life of foods.

Cumin: the second-most popular herb in the world after black pepper, has a distinct pleasant taste, used in Mexican and Spanish dishes, mostly for tacos and chili; helps digestion and provides essential minerals including phosphorus, thiamine, and potassium.

Mints: mostly peppermint and spearmint leaves are used as teas, but can be added to meats and desserts; are found in breath fresheners and toothpastes and can calm digestive problems and alleviate nausea.

Oregano: a common ingredient in Italian and Greek cuisine, best sprinkled on savory food and added to soups; antiviral, antibacterial, antibiotic, and high in antioxidants.

Rosemary: has a pine-lemony scent and is used mostly in lamb dishes, vegetables and soups; adds years to your life by rejuvenating the small blood vessels under the skin.

Sage: can be added to most any dish and in turkey, chicken, or pork chop stuffing; has antioxidant and anti-inflammatory effects, improves memory, and lengthens life.

Thyme: mostly used in French and Italian cooking and when added at the start of baked dishes will slowly release its benefits; as thyme water it can be used as a mouthwash or taken internally to speed an illness recovery.

Turmeric: a common ingredient in Indian foods—chutney and curries—and adds a spark of flavor to soups, meats, sauces, and baked foods; its key component, curcumin, is a powerful anti-inflammatory and an effective pain reliever.

All herbs and spices are derived from plants: flowers, fruits, seeds, barks, and roots—offering many health benefits but without any calories. Others you may consider adding to your culinary creations include garlic, parsley, arrowroot, cloves, ginger, nutmeg, saffron, cilantro, ginseng, cardamom, and fennel. However, before increasing your collection, confer with your health professional, since some, like ginger, turmeric, peppermint oil, and others, have qualities that may not be compatible with a medical condition you have.

Enjoy the benefits and exciting flavors of herbs and spices
but make sure to check the expiration dates
to maintain their nutritional value.

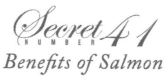

Benefits of Salmon

Enjoy delectable plank-grilled salmon.

During my college years, 1938 to 1942, we were served home-style meals in huge and inviting dining halls. The food was prepared by a master chef and was always good and sometimes great, and we were able to enjoy the campus custom of mingling with classmates during mealtime. However, many students skipped Friday dinners for one simple reason: Friday was fish night. Seafood, at that time, was cheap but never a favorite. Over the years, university dining has changed to small fast food facilities, and fish has become an accepted delicious, nutritious super food, with a corresponding increase in cost. Salmon ranks high among all species for its nutritional benefits. It is an outstanding source of minerals and vitamins, including selenium, vitamin B12, and potassium. Beyond these benefits, salmon receives extra high points for its content of omega-3 fatty acids.

There are many types of salmon, and researchers continue to find more benefits in all of them and anticipate discovering more. Among those recommended most often is wild Alaskan salmon. No matter which type you prefer, salmon can be prepared in several different ways. I offer a favorite recipe here that I found on WebMD. Try it? It's delectable!

Plank-Grilled Salmon

Ingredients for four servings:

4 5-ounce fillets/steaks wild salmon, 3/4"–1" thick sodium

1/4 cup soy sauce, reduced

1/4 cup sake or dry white wine

1/4 cup mirin

3 tablespoon coarsely chopped fresh ginger

2 tablespoons sugar

3 tablespoons coarsely chopped scallions.

1 small onion, thinly sliced

Directions:

Step 1: Soak a grilling plank in water for 2 to 4 hours.

Step 2: Combine soy sauce, sake, or white wine, mirin, sugar, scallions, and ginger in a small saucepan and bring to a boil. Remove from heat and cool to room temperature.

Step 3: Place salmon in a shallow dish and pour the marinade over it. Place lemon slices on top. Marinate in refrigerator at least 30 minutes, no more than 2 hours. Turn fish once or twice.

Step 4: Preheat grill to medium high.

Step 5: Place the plank over direct heat on the grill and heat for 2 minutes. Move the plank so it is over indirect heat. Remove the salmon from the marinade, place it skin side down on the hot plank and replace the lemon slices on top. Close the lid and cook until the fish is just cooked through, 10 to 15 minutes. You may use the plank as the serving platter.

Serve with veggies, a salad and a glass of wine! Bon appétit!

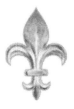

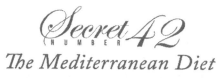

Secret Number 42
The Mediterranean Diet
The cuisine of the people of the Mediterranean

One day recently as I was browsing the Internet, I happened upon the Mediterranean diet. Though I have been aware of this food movement, I have never pursued it in depth. To my surprise, I learned that the recommended fare is what I have been cooking and eating most of my life. If you already know all about this diet and its benefits, move on to my next Secret. Otherwise, read on and learn about this extraordinarily basic diet, which studies show can maintain or even increase the size of your brain (which can decrease in volume as time passes) and may add years to your life.

What is a Mediterranean diet?

The Mediterranean is not a traditional diet—it is not created for the sole purpose of weight loss. It is a group of foods consumed by the people of France, Italy, Greece, Spain, and the Middle East.

What are the foods in Mediterranean cuisine? They include: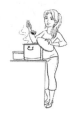

Fresh fruit: Include three to four pieces of fresh fruit and some berries in your meals and snacks every day. They are high in antioxidants that protect against diseases.

Whole grains: Only eat whole wheat or whole-grain breads. Have whole wheat pasta two or three times a week.

Legumes: Eat two to four cups of cooked legumes—dried beans, lentils, peas, garbanzo beans—two or three times a week.

Veggies: Have a salad with olive oil and lemon for dressing at dinner time. Be sure to include a tomato, a staple Mediterranean veggie. Sauté green beans, zucchini, or another veggie in olive oil and garlic for a side dish. Delicious.

Nuts: Enjoy a quarter cup of nuts—almonds and walnuts are the healthiest—for a morning or afternoon break. Nuts are high in monounsaturated fats.

Fish and seafood: Two to three servings of fish are a must every week. Salmon and sardines are top choices, since they offer high levels of Omega-3 oils.

Olive oil: Substitute olive oil for butter or other fats for cooking and condiments. Use olive oil for a dip for whole-grain breads.

Aromatic herbs and garlic: Replace salt and condiments with aromatic herbs and garlic.

Other: Limit red meat to only one serving a month; replace sugar with honey and avoid all processed foods.

Benefits of Mediterranean foods:

Researchers, including Yian Gu, assistant professor of neuropsychology at Columbia University in New York City, agree that studies show that the Mediterranean diet is a healthy diet with benefits that

- make your brain the equivalent of five years younger
- improve your cognitive capacity
- lower the risk of breast cancer and heart disease
- can keep depression at bay and in some cases cure the condition
- lengthen your life expectancy

After pursuing the research on Mediterranean foods, I began to realize that this diet has contributed largely to my living a healthy long life. If you wish to enjoy its benefits, check with your doctor or health professional to learn if you can start now and add years to your life.

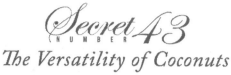

Secret 43
The Versatility of Coconuts

Coconut oil has always been a staple in tropical countries, especially in India, Thailand, the Philippines, Burma, coastal Africa, and Sri Lanka. After being maligned during the 1970s in the United States and Canada the oil has rebounded with acknowledged extensive benefits. The corn and soy oil industry claimed coconut oil was harmful because of its saturated oil content. Not so!

Coconut oil proponents—among them scientists, nutritionists, and alternative medicine practitioners—assert that "different types of saturated fats behave differently in the body and that lauric acid, the principal saturated fat in coconut oil, increases the levels of HDL 'good' cholesterol as well LD, 'bad' cholesterol."

Further, the Coconut Research Center has released studies that show coconut oil has traces of unsaturated fatty acids including capric acid, caprylic acid, and lauric acid that contribute to its numerous benefits. It is now being heralded as a miracle cure for a wide range of ailments, a weight-loss and longevity booster, and a nondairy substitute for butter.

Types of coconut oil include pure coconut oil, virgin coconut oil, refined coconut oil, organic coconut oil, and organic virgin coconut oil.

If you choose to use coconut oil, it is wise to determine why you want to and how and which type to use. You may ask your professional health adviser which will meet your needs. Here are the basic uses:

Good health: virgin coconut oil and organic coconut oil
Cooking: refined coconut oil
Weight loss: virgin coconut oil
Skin care and massaging: pure coconut oil, refined coconut oil
Hair care: pure coconut oil, refined coconut oil
Medicinal uses: virgin coconut oil, organic virgin coconut oil

You might want to try two other products of the coconut. Its milk sipped through a straw from the coconut is a delightful, refreshing drink. When you have emptied the coconut make sure you enjoy its pure white meat.

In the next Secret I discuss the boundless benefits of coconut oil.

Secret Number 44
The Benefits of Coconut Oil

The uses of coconut oil go beyond serving as an effective substitute for butter and other oils in cooking, baking, and salads. It has internal and external uses that contribute to its long list of health benefits. Its unique combination of fatty acids have profound positive effects on our health. These acids—caprylic, capric, myristic, lauric, linoleic, oleic, palmitic, and stearic—give coconut oil antimicrobial, antiviral, antioxidant, antifungal, and other powerful medicinal properties. Coconut oil has been confirmed in human studies as one of the few that can be classified as a "superfood"!

*Here are some of the proven benefits of coconut oil
according to studies by the Coconut Research Center:*

Health benefits: Lauric acid in coconut oil helps kill bacteria, viruses, and fungi and staves off infections. The oil also strengthens the immune system, improves bone health, prevents and treats diseases, and lessens symptoms of stress.

Weight control: Coconut oil reduces your appetite and raises the metabolic rate, which boosts energy and endurance and helps burn fat, contributing to the loss of body weight.

Dental health: Coconut oil, when used as a mouth wash, kills harmful bacteria in the mouth, improves dental health and reduces bad breath.

Skin care: Coconut oil is a superb skin moisturizer, acting as a sunscreen to block out 20 percent of the sun's ultraviolet rays. It helps avoid premature signs of aging by preventing wrinkles, sagging skin, skin dryness, flaking damaged skin, chapped lips and cold sores. Wow!

Hair care: Coconut oil is used to treat dry and damaged hair and as a lathering ingredient in soaps and shampoos. It encourages healthy growth and gives hair a shiny glow.

I have long been aware of the importance of coconut oil, but after pursuing my research, I am now convinced that it is indeed, a miracle cure.

You, too, can enjoy the benefits of coconut oil
and add years to your life!

IX. Running

Secret *45*
(NUMBER)

The Pluses of a Five-Minute-a-Day Run

Though the Centers for Disease Control and Prevention recommend that adults exercise at least one hour and fifteen minutes a week doing an aerobic physical activity at a vigorous level, only 5 percent of Americans have a daily exercise regimen. By running just five minutes a day you can enjoy several life-extending benefits. Or if you are one of the many to whom running does not appeal, you can walk briskly for 15 minutes a day and reap the same benefits. I've been enjoying them for many years

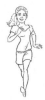

I walk briskly at least a mile-and a half each morning with Niqui, my gentle Whippet, and I practice exercises prescribed by Jen, my trainer, for a half hour late in the day. I also have two half-hour sessions with her each week!

The Benefits of Running

When you choose to engage in at least two hours and thirty minutes of aerobic physical activity at a moderate level each week, you will meet the requirements that ensure healthful benefits. Here they are as reported in various medical journals, along with how running or walking will enhance them:

Your mood: Running will boost your spirits and put you in a good frame of mind. Many runners declare they get a "runner's high" after the end of a good run. Practicing an intense endurance activity can increase your endocannabinoids, the brain chemicals that indicate pleasure.

Your sleep: A daily morning run can help you get a good night's sleep. It will improve objective sleep and the quality and mood of subjective sleep and concentration during the day.

Your blood pressure: According to the American Heart Association, running or brisk walking can lower the risk of high blood pressure, high cholesterol, and diabetes.

Your brain: Running or walking as your regular daily exercise can raise your heart rate and increase the flow of oxygen-rich blood in your body, as well as to your brain.

Your heart: A run of only five minutes a day can cut the risk of cardiovascular disease almost in half. If you run regularly you have a 30 percent lower risk of dying from all causes and a remarkable 45percent lower risk of death from cardiovascular disease.

Your life span: Five minutes a day will keep the doctor away, and best of all your life span will extend at least six years.

Run! Walk briskly!
Enjoy the benefits and add years to your life.

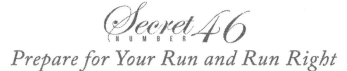

Prepare for Your Run and Run Right

Want to enjoy the benefits of running as discussed in Secret 45? If you are not properly prepared and do not develop correct running form, you may not only miss out on achieving the benefits and a "runner's high" but you may do harm to parts of your body. Patrick Murphy, a trainer for celebrities, has some suggestions that will ensure you start your runs on the right foot. Murphy says that running properly is a "super mood booster as well as an efficient calorie-burner."

How to prepare for your runs:

Exercise to prevent injury: Regularly practice the 100 ups, known as "high knees" which is like running in place. Stand with your feet hip-width apart. Drive your right knee forward toward your chest and quickly place it back on the ground.

Repeat with your left knee.   Do 100 high knees, 50 more slowly, then another set of 50 double time.

Proper shoes: Do not run in everyday sneakers. Get the best fit you can at a legitimate running shoe store.

Find a partner or group: Like-minded runners will keep you motivated and consistent.

Make progress slowly: Start with a walk, then run a short distance. Increase both over a given period of time and you will avoid injuries.

Don't run on a full or empty stomach: Eat a whole apple or orange before you start your run to give you a boost. They are low in calories and easy to digest. Do the same after your run until you cool down.

These preps will ensure your runs are successful.

How to run right—make sure you develop your best running form!
(tips from Personal Best Training and Fitness Programs)

First: As you run, focus on your body, feel how you use your muscles and move your frame.

Second: Relax. Keep your shoulders, face, and hands as loose and free as possible, with your hands close to your waist.

Third: Shift your weight as you go up hills. Lift your arms slightly to raise your center of gravity.

Fourth: Touch the ground lightly. To do so, listen to the sound you make as your shoes hit the pavement. Adjust as necessary to lighten the sound.

You can prepare for your runs and develop a good running form on your own. But if you are not sure you are running right, call on a trainer at a YMCA/YWCA or a wellness center for guidance.

Enjoy your "runner's high"!

Secret Number 47
The Draw and Dangers of Treadmills

It looks so easy to run in place on a treadmill! And I can tell you it is, once you have learned how. And if you prepare properly and run right (as reviewed in Secrets 45 and 46). you will enjoy benefits and advantages similar to those of ground running and more. You can move at your own pace and imagine you are on a tree-lined street in a country village. However, you must be aware of the risks and how to handle them.

Before I discuss the risks, I offer some of the up sides of working out on a treadmill.

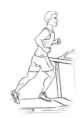

First: The surface of a treadmill is uniform and easier to maneuver than sidewalks, potholed roads, and uneven trails.

Second: You can customize your program to suit the time you have to exercise.

Third: A treadmill is easy to operate. You control your speed, incline, energy spent, and warm-up and cool-down sessions.

Fourth: Your treadmill is available inside so you can run even during inclement weather.

Fifth: Generally, treadmill running burns calories faster than other exercise methods.

Disadvantages of treadmill exercising

Despite the advantages treadmills offer, I find that standing in place on one in the same surroundings for any length of time can be boring. Though you can watch television or listen to an audio, I choose other exercises that involve more parts of my body. Also, treadmills are limited to walking and running. More importantly, according to the Sports and Fitness Industry Association, "exercise equipment and treadmills in particular, can be dangerous." Every year, thousands of Americans are injured on these machines.

How to Use a Treadmill Safely

Here are a few treadmill safety suggestions from physiologist Mike Bracko of Calgary, Alberta, who has written a guide on the proper use of treadmills:

- Avoid using your phone on a treadmill. Phones are major distractions that can cause you to trip and fall.

- Clip the emergency stop mechanism to your shirt or pants. Straddle the treadmill with your feet on the rubber strips that are on either side of the belt. Hit the "Quickstart" to get the treadmill going at a slow pace, .5 or 1 mph.

- Start walking on the treadmill, keeping the pace slow until you are comfortable. Then, very gradually increase it until you are walking moderately. Later, you may move on to running.

- Getting off: Slow down the treadmill gradually, almost to a stop. Do not stop abruptly, for you may lose your balance. And never get off a rapidly moving treadmill. When the treadmill is moving at its slowest pace, hold the handrails and place one foot at a time on the rubber strips, so that you are straddling the belt. Hit stop and unclip the emergency devise. Turn around and walk off on the rubber strips, not the belt.

Once you have mastered these cautionary measures
you will be able to enjoy the benefits and advantages
of the most popular type of exercise equipment in America.
(Even though I get bored!)

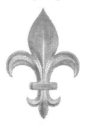

X. Take Time Out to Relax

Secret 48
(NUMBER)

Enjoy Your Holidays

Practicing a yoga pose will help you relax and prepare you to make the most of the holidays. You deserve to take a break from your regular tasks. One of the easiest and most restorative yoga postures is the Child's Pose—*Balasana*. A couple of caveats: You may enroll in a class at a studio or have private lessons with a trainer to help you carry out the postures correctly and avoid injury before you do them on your own. And check with your doctor to make sure you are in sound physical condition to handle the routines safely.

To prepare for practicing any yoga pose, see Secrets 24 and 25!

Balasana is a soothing posture that relieves the tension in the lower back and neck and the tightness in your shoulder blades. This pose is calming and stretches the legs, ankles, thighs, hips, knees, and back muscles. It is also wonderful for the stomach and aids digestion by gently stimulating the stomach and lower bowel.

Step 1: Start by sitting upright on your knees, keeping them wide apart. Keep your feet together, big toes touching, your fanny resting on your heel and your palms down.

Step 2: Breathe, inhaling deeply. While exhaling, bring your chest down between your knees and swing your arms forward in front of you and place your forehead on the mat.

Step 3: Bring your arms back to your sides and rest your hands palms up on either side of your feet.

Step 4: Take four deep, conscious breaths as you hold the Child's Pose.

Step 5: Return to the upright kneeling position with your back straight and your hands on your thighs.

Step 6: Repeat this pose two or three times.

Now you should be ready to relax and enjoy the holidays. Welcome them with joy, optimism, and an open mind. However, if you don't choose to do the Child's Pose now, don't. But schedule a practice for sometime throughout the year.

Secret Number 49

A Day at the Spa Once a Year

Indulging in a day to relax and be pampered at a spa goes beyond what we all deserve and will help add years to your life. However, it is wise to be cautious and selective. Take time to understand the services to ensure you will experience those that benefit you most, and what you can afford. You will find many spas on the Internet with a variety of price ranges. Once you have made your decision, check with your doctor to make sure you are physically fit for your day, or longer, at the spa.

Selecting the spa that's right for you

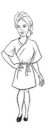

A good way to start is to ask your friends for suggestions and to contact spas for references from some of their guests. Try to make time for a visit. It will be easier to check the cleanliness and tidiness, the friendliness of management and staff, that the type of services offered are those you seek, and that the technicians are certified and the products they use are high in quality.

Some typical spa therapies

Spa retreats are usually beautiful resorts in stunning settings, with handsome buildings and designer suites, all that immediately put you in a mood to recharge, rejuvenate, and reenergize. You can arrange your schedule of treatments from many: a sauna, a massage, a facial, a manicure, a pedicure, hair styling, a body wrap, acupuncture, detoxing, and a variety of lectures on nutrition and healthy living. There are fun fitness activities of hiking, swimming, tennis, Pilates, and even boxing. Along with delectable, good-for-you gourmet meals, there are times for naps and restful night sleeping. Everything is designed to pamper you, help you relax, and have the time of your life, even if it is only for a day.

You deserve to benefit from a day at a spa at least once a year.
Even better try two or three or extend your stay to a week.
If you're on a budget, even a morning, an afternoon, or an hour
will give you a lift.

Secret 50

Select Spa Therapies That Are Best For You

Once you have arrived at your spa of choice, one that has been highly recommended and safe, you can settle in to relax and be pampered. A great way to start is to get to know the staff and the other guests and explore the elegant public areas. Then stroll the paths through magnificent gardens and follow with a healthful gourmet lunch. You may take a nap on the patio or in your designer suite before you meet with an expert planner to develop your schedule of exercise and therapy treatments that will help you reenergize and recharge.

Here are some therapies you can select from.
All have many benefits. I mention a few.

Body wraps: This treatment is best for you if you want to lose weight. All or parts of your body are covered with seaweed or mud and then wrapped with bandages and a heated blanket. You rest for forty-five minutes, remove the wrappings, and shower. There are several types of body wraps for a variety of benefits, including replenishing your body with nutrients and boosting moisture in your skin.

Massages: Massage technicians manipulate their fingers to relax muscle tension in your back, shoulders, neck, legs, and head. Craniosacral therapy relaxes the soft tissues surrounding your central nervous system. The numerous types of massage and their benefits place your mind, body, and spirit in harmony.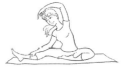

Detoxing with an ionic footbath: Ionic footbath has many benefits, from enhancing your immune system to improving your liver and kidney functions. It sends a small current that goes in a circuit through the body, generating positively charged ions. They neutralize the toxins so the body can discard them through the pores of your feet and correct the PH balance in your body. Many spas offer other methods of detoxing.

Acupuncture: The practice of acupuncture is designed to restore the body's balance, eliminate pain, and improve sleep. The procedure is done by thrusting, plucking, and vibrating needles in select parts of the body. This Chinese technique has been accepted as effective by Western scientists.

Facials and make up: Facial treatments correct hyperpigmentation and uneven skin tones, repair collagen and elastin, and improve and brighten your skin. You have a choice of subtle or bold make up, and you will be shown how to do it yourself.

Manicure/pedicure: Your fingernails and toenails will be painted and polished to perfection. Your hands and arms will be treated to a warm cream massage, as well as your feet and lower legs.

Sauna baths: According to a feature in the Journal of the America Medical Association, sitting in a superheated room and perspiring profusely on a regular basis can help you live longer. The finding is based on results from a Finnish study of almost 2,500 men. The rooms were heated to 174 degrees Fahrenheit.

These brief descriptions of a few therapies spas offer should help you find in-depth information in books and libraries and on the Internet to determine your choices.

Again, I recommend you spend a day, a week, an hour at the spa,
whatever you have time for and can afford.
You will add years to your life!

Secret 51

Indulge In a Be Kind To Me Day
One every month will extend your life.

Early in my career when I was a fashion editor at Woman's Day magazine, a colleague, Nancy, arrived at the office looking fresher and more vibrant than usual. I was surprised, since she had a trying photo shoot that day with our Devil Wears Prada–type boss. Sensing my surprise, Nancy, with a lilt in her voice, said, "Oh, yesterday was my 'Be kind to Nancy day.' I'm ready for whatever the 'Witch of Seventh Avenue' dishes out."

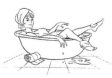 All due respect to MPG, our Fashion Editor—she was a brilliant, informed style maven, a hard-driving no-nonsense woman. She knew how to spot and promote the best classic style trends. MPG had her hang ups, however, and did not hesitate to take them out on her staff, including me.

Nevertheless, I owe her much. I learned design, style, and the whims of the fashion world. She taught me to trust my instincts. She'd ask my opinion and subtly credited me for good taste, which up to then I didn't know I had.

But that day, it was from Nancy that I learned an important lesson that has helped me countless times since—how to prepare for an anticipated session of verbal abuse or other difficult situations: Pamper yourself for a day! You will add years to your life!

Page 59

Here are some tips to help you design your Be Kind to Me Day

Sleep late: Once you are up, take a hot bath and soak till the water cools or add more hot water. Once out of the tub, slip into a comfortable robe, schlep around your home, relax in a plush chair with a cup of coffee or tea and read your paper.

Pig out: Indulge in the forbidden foods you've stocked in your fridge and pantry or have brunch at a fast food place. For dinner, treat yourself to a gourmet meal at a French, Italian, Chinese, Thai, or other favorite restaurants. Be sure to include a glass of wine or two and a big dessert.

Spend the afternoon at something you've wanted to or ought to do: a shopping spree, a walk on a nature trail, a drive along peaceful country roads, a swim at the local Y; volunteer at the community charity or visit a salon or spa for a facial, hairdo, or massage; stay at home and read a book; watch a soap opera or a film; take a nap; or whatever turns you on.

Your evening is to entertain you: Attend the theater, a concert, the opera, or a sports event or just go to bed early and watch television till you fall asleep. Avoid the news—it's too depressing.

Your Be Kind To Me Day
will help you handle challenges, refreshed and restored—
and add years to your life.
Be Kind to You. It's your day!

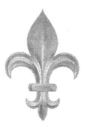

Secret 52
It's Not About How You Look—
It's How You Feel!

But looking good can make you feel great!

When I was in my eighties my friends began to ask what my secret was for looking younger. It wasn't until I turned ninety that I came to acknowledge that I am living a healthy, happy, sexy, long life. What is the reason for that? It's simple: I do everything possible to make sure that I always feel good—or great. I am told that I look and act about sixty though I feel even younger.

My friends see the outer me, I feel and measure the inner me—and that along with practicing my Secrets makes me appear much younger because I'm happy and healthy. There are many of my friends who say they reflect the inner me when we spend time together, and they feel good about themselves. That makes me feel even better.

What does feeling good really mean?

Feeling good is not just that you are happy: it is a message from your inner being telling you that you are on the right track. The universal source of energy is letting you know you are going in the proper direction and informing you on how to proceed.

Reasons why you should feel good

There is nothing more important than feeling good. Feeling bad is an indication that you are on the wrong path either physically, spiritually, or personally. Feeling good opens doors to explore new experiences, expand relationships, get creative juices flowing, be more creative, become more confident, achieve goals more quickly, and feel motivated to take part in activities that improve your health and help you savor the best things in life.

Ways to make yourself feel good

The best ways to make yourself feel good are those that make you happy, smile, and laugh. Surround yourself only with people who are feeling good about themselves. Spend more time with someone you love and who loves you. Acknowledge and appreciate the good things that happen to you. Listen to music that you enjoy and gives you a lift. Tell yourself that you want to feel good or feel better. Say it again and again until you do.

Look in the mirror and smile. You will look great and feel good!

Never forget that one of the best ways to make yourself feel good
is to take a walk in nature and smell the flowers.

Secret № 53
How to Beat That Overtired Feeling

Ways you can boost your energy:
build an arsenal of basic positive strategies

Almost everyone I know feels they are so busy that when night falls they are exhausted. Every once in a while, I experience much the same, since I have set goals with a time schedule that I am hard pressed to achieve. To avoid fatigue, I make sure I accomplish as much as possible each day, am satisfied with the progress I have made, and am in bed at a reasonable hour. I aim to refrain from overloading my body and my mind to avoid being overtired. It takes dedication and practicing energy strategies.

If your fatigue is due to a health problem or a disease, it is important that you discuss your situation with your health-care provider. Most non-health-related overtiredness is caused by heavy workloads and long hours without breaks. You can boost your energy levels with a regimen of positive strategies.

Here are some energy boosters

1. Learn your energy levels. Observe them and schedule demanding projects when you are at your energy peak.

2. Cut back on the amount of news you watch, read about, and listen to. Most news is negative and depressing.

3. Take fifteen minutes out of your work day for a walk in nature.

4. Develop a healthy diet, drink lots of water, have breakfast every day, and take a daily dose of Omega-3 fish oil.

5. Try some golden root. Rhodiola Rosea is an adaptogen that reduces symptoms of stress, improves mental stability, and more.

6. At night, take a bath in sea salt and make a habit of retiring early.

7. Listen to classical music.

8. Surround yourself with happy, positive people.

9. When a negative incident happens in your life that is responsible for your overtired feeling, turn around; do something positive—a good deed for a friend, or a special indulgence for yourself.

You needn't perform all these energy boosters, just enough to make a difference and overcome that overtired feeling. Experiment with two or three at a time to learn which help the most. For those that may impact your health, check with your health-care provider to determine which boosters are best for you. Once you have found those you can rely on, make them daily habits. You will feel improvement in creativity, concentration, performance, and overall health. You deserve to be free of fatigue, be energized, and add years to your life.

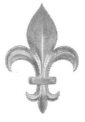

XI. Friendships

Secret NUMBER 54

The Art of Nonsexual Touching and the Hug

Try it, you'll like it!

I am a hugger! I am not alone. The French, Italians, Greeks, and most Europeans are generous with their physical affection. But few Americans do it. However, you will see joyful athletes throughout our country on the playing fields spontaneously hug in groups and do "high fives" after a score or a victory.

I suggest you try it and enjoy the healing powers of the touch! I spread the practice to new friends as we part. My old ones know what to expect and I meet no resistance from them or from the new. They happily accept my hugs and return them in kind.

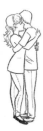 There has not been a lot of research on the topic of interpersonal touch. However, here is some advice from an expert. "Don't limit the number of hugs you give," suggests Virginia Satir, a noted twentieth-century family therapist. "We need four hugs a day for survival. We need eight hugs a day for maintenance. We need twelve hugs a day for growth."

Enjoy the benefits of touch

Despite the limited research, studies show there is a sense of feel-good energy from a hug, a handshake, a cuddle, a snuggle, holding hands, or even a pat on the back, all given in a healthy way. Here are some of the benefits you will experience when you touch:

• When you start with a friendly, affectionate touch, your body releases oxytocin, often called the love hormone, lowering blood pressure and decreasing the stress-related hormone cortisol. Feelings of loneliness, isolation, and anger can disappear.

• Hugging reminds our bodies of the cuddling we received in our early years and connects us to self-love.

• The feelings brought about by hugs can build trust and a sense of safety that will open sincere communication.

• Maintaining a hug for a few moments raises the serotonin levels, lifts your mood, and helps you feel happiness.

• The immune system is strengthened by touching. Research proves that the thymus gland, which regulates and balances the body's production of white blood cells, is stimulated to keep us healthy and disease free.

• Any touching will help secure a relationship. It encourages understanding and empathy and confirms your friendship or love.

There's more! Research reveals that petting your dog or cat, even giving your horse a hug, will lower your blood pressure and help relieve your stress. However, Bonnie Beaver, professor of animal behavior at the College of Veterinary Medicine, Texas A&M University, says, "It's more significant if the pet is your own. Otherwise, there's tension: 'Is this one going to bite me?'" Again, the benefits are due to the release of oxytocin, also acknowledged as a calming hormone.

So touch . . . your family members, your friends, **and** *your pets!*

Secret 55

Good Friends Add Years to Your Life

Close, sincere relationships with family members and friends are assurance that we will live more fulfilling and longer lives. We have a need for these bonds, which are among the most critical aspects of human existence—relating to and interacting with others. Friends we have made in every period of our lives from early childhood through the mature years have lasting effects on how we live. These influences are subtle, and most often we are unaware of how they may have affected us. Also, each of us has had at least one friend or mentor who has put us on a path that has dramatically changed our lives.

The importance of friends in your life

• Meeting with friends can be an escape from the stress of today's high-pressured living where you will experience laughter, fun, joy, and happiness.

- Spending time together can be inspirational.

- You can turn to friends in difficult times or good times for support and guidance.

- A glass of wine or a beer with a friend will help you relax. (Just don't overimbibe. You can always share a pot of tea instead.)

- You can count on friends for encouragement when you undertake a challenging project.

- Friends can help you feel your inner strength, your courage, and your self-image.

- Over a period of time, you may develop a business relationship or volunteer or do fund-raising projects for your community.

- You can develop at least one very special friend to whom you can turn to help you through a loss, a tragedy, or any overwhelming experience.

Treasure your friends. Hear what they have to say. Nurture them and they will nurture you in return. Be there for them when they need you and they will be there for you for your needs. You both will benefit and together you will share happy, rewarding, long lives. And don't neglect cultivating new friends.

Secret 56
Build a Roster of Diverse Friendships

Most of us are inclined to select and attract friends who are much like us with similar interests—those in whom we see our own image. It is easy and safe to fall into and remain in this pattern. However, according to Dr. Suzy Green, clinical and coaching psychologist and founder of the Positive Institute, "It is important to have a diversity of friends to be able to look for support from a variety of sources." She goes on to say, "They also help us keep a broader perspective on life."

From the time I was a child I have gravitated to people with talents, professions, interests, ages, ethnicities, objectives, and accomplishments different from mine. They have enriched and nourished my life and gratified my restless curiosity, which continues as I mature. (Note that I do not say "age.")

I write here about three I have befriended recently. I've just added a fourteen-year-young girl who is a tech geek to my list. She helps me increase my knowledge of current advances in technology. Another recent addition is my marketing guru—a thirty-eight-year-old Trinidadian American who is also a brilliant computer expert and former film stunt man. He works out of Arizona and has a lovely wife and four little kids. Though we have yet to meet, we have become more than friends. We are family.

The third is Mary Hartman, whom I met several years ago when she was dean of my college, Douglass, and I was an alumna volunteer. Though she is two decades younger than I, I have great respect for her and consider her my role model. More recently, at a fund-raiser at my home for the institute she founded at Rutgers University, she told the donors in her talk that I was her role model. Quite a surprise!

You never know what great things lie in store for you
when you have diverse friends.

To help you seek out types of diverse friends that can help you enjoy a happy long life, I offer a few suggestions of what to look for from Domonique Bertolucci, a life coach and author of The Happiness Code:

The friend who is cooler than you: The people who are current and up to date, the beacons of cool. They enrich your life with things that may have passed you by.

The friend who is up for anything: These are friends you can call on anytime, for any reason, at the drop of a hat. They are flexible, open to new things, and will change plans at short notice.

The friend you aspire to be: The friends who lift you higher. They see the best in you and give you feedback on your strength and weaknesses.

The friend who doesn't know any of your other friends: A friend who is not involved and can offer objective advice. There is a level of privacy in this friendship that doesn't exist in circles of friends.

The friend who is painfully honest: This friend will not always tell you what you want to hear. He or she will tell you what you need to know, with good intentions and for your benefit.

The friend who knows you better than you know yourself: This friend has known you since you were still in diapers. He or she knows you out of the context of your growing up, your schooling, your work, and your relationships and accepts you for who you are.

When you find people who have any of these traits, cherish them and add them to your roster of diverse friends. They will nourish, enrich, and add years to your life.

Secret 57
Communicate Face to Face

I don't go as far back as the days of the Pony Express or even to the introduction of the telegraph. However, when I was a four-year-old girl, I clearly remember that telephones were in their infancy and that few could afford the newfangled device that provided instant communication. If you could afford one, you'd share a party line and often listen in on a neighbor's conversation. I also recall the early days when radio was considered a miracle and television was still years away.

Most communication was handwritten and traveled days by mail to its destination. Or you would visit friends or family, sit down at the kitchen table or in a cozy living room for a pleasant (or unpleasant) face-to-face chat. Business communication was handled much the same way—with personal meetings in offices to resolve critical issues. However, in large cities, business mail could be delivered in minutes by messenger on bicycle.

In today's world, the personal exchange has all but disappeared and technology has taken over. We have come to expect and rely on the convenient, instant contact of e-mail, texting, Facebook, Twitter, Instagram, and cell phones. Yet we are often frustrated when our message fails to get through within moments.

Nonetheless, there are times when we do arrange face-to-face communication, by choice, emergency, or necessity. Refreshing! When we do, there is a sense of understanding before a word is uttered. A handshake, a hug, or body language can be as loud as a shout. Clear meaning is also transmitted in your tone, the inflection of your voice, your facial expression, and through hard-to-hide emotions.

A meeting in person demonstrates the importance of the message, gets the attention of your audience, helps you see and be able to respond quickly to the listener's reactions, permits you to address sensitive issues more easily, and helps address and handle them quickly.

You will find that increasing your number of face-to-face encounters
will not only help you "close more deals"
they will divert you from your stressful tech pace
and add years to your life!

XII. Brain Power

Secret Number 58
Build a Healthier, Sharper Brain

Starting early in your career by taking on a challenging job can help protect and improve your brain power and add years to your life. A recent study of more than a thousand people over seventy-five, published in the journal Neurology, reported that those who had held jobs that required performing complicated tasks had half the rate of cognitive decline of those whose jobs were less demanding. The tasks include those that require concentrated mental effort, full and close attention, resolving conflicts, analyzing data, and taking on new and different projects.

Even if you are in your sixties or seventies it's not too late to begin.

The old adage "you can't teach an old dog new tricks" has been proven obsolete. According to scientific studies, the ability of the brain to adapt to change, known as neuroplasticity, is astonishing. My family and many of my friends (all much younger than I) are amazed at how I continue to learn, put my new knowledge to work, and help others by researching and writing my Secrets (even as I keep on living them).

Are you comfortable with the performance of your brain at your job and with your other everyday activities? If you aren't, it's time for a mental workout. The sooner you start undertaking mental challenges, the more you are assured of developing a healthier, sharper brain as you mature. Try something new. Learn a new language or to play a musical instrument. Take a class in pottery, painting, sculpture, psychology, dancing—or something you always wanted to do or explore but have put off.

When you accept the challenge, you will enjoy unexpected rewards, build a healthier, sharper brain, and extend the length of your life.

Secret Number 59
Preserve and Enhance Your Memory

As we grow and mature into adults, not only does our brain retain the power to improve our learning abilities and absorb new information, it can enhance our memory no matter how young or mature (old) we might be. However, you cannot leave moving forward to chance. You have to call on memory-enhancing techniques for help. They are not the fun, much-touted brain games. Research has shown that these amusing pastimes, even with daily practice, do little to boost your brain. They might result in short-term improvements in the specific game category. But they do not last or work long term to strengthen your memory or help you learn information and retain it.

Not to worry. There are many ways to improve your memory
and some that you will enjoy.

We humans are social animals. Our brains respond to and are stimulated by interaction with others. Once you accept socializing as an important part of your life, you will benefit from the basic, proven methods that boost your brain. Start by committing yourself to practicing at least one at a time. Once you have conquered the first and it becomes a part of your subconscious, move on to another. Here are a few mental exercises that are worth trying:

Pay attention: Don't just listen to something of lasting interest; hear it and store it away in your brain.

Repeat: Repetition is the simplest, easiest way to retain information. Repeat, repeat, repeat, not just once but several times when you first hear a name, a place, a title, a street, a town, a phone number—whatever you want to remember.

Organize: Keeping a day planner, making to-do lists, taking notes, organizing information, and jotting down conversations, events, and thoughts are all helpful techniques. I keep a journal every night of what I accomplished during the day. I'm prepared and fresh to start the next morning.

Rhymes: Call up well-known rhymes, poetry, or songs you already know or create your own as reminders. My favorite that I learned when I was a little girl:

Thirty days hath September, April June and November,
All the rest have thirty-one, excepting February alone,
Which has eight and a score till leap year gives it one more.

Acronyms (or something close): The first letters of a phrase or group used to help remember it. Recently, my exercise trainer helped me remember and differentiate between two similar exercises among scores I already know: TUSSS, for Toes Up, Stand Straight Stretch. FFBB for Feet Flat, Butt Back. How can I forget?

There are several other worthwhile methods like involving your senses, visualizing, chunking, and acrostics. However, winning takes work. If you regularly practice some of the above, you will enhance your memory and add years to your life.

Secret 60

Exercise, the Brain Power Booster

No one will deny that exercising the brain by practicing mental gymnastics helps to keep your mind fit. Referenced by scientific studies as "neurobics," these practices "engage our attention to stand out from everyday activities as unusual, fun, surprising and can even evoke emotions like happiness, love or anger." They also strengthen nerve connections and activate little-used pathways in your brain.

However, few people know or accept that physical exercise contributes much to boost the brain by protecting the memory and improving thinking skills. According to a report in the Harvard Health Letter, physical activity can reduce insulin resistance, decrease inflammation, and stimulate the release of growth factors—chemicals in the brain that can increase the number of new blood vessels as well as brain cells and improve their survival.

Regular aerobic exercise, which gets your heart and sweat glands pumping, has been found to boost the size of the hippocampus, the area of the brain that is involved with verbal memory and learning. Brisk walking for an hour twice a week is another beneficial exercise. Or try other moderate physical activities for ten or fifteen minutes every day. Other things like swimming, tennis, volleyball, or dancing also count. Even household chores such as heavy floor mopping, raking leaves, or whatever gets your heart going so you break out in a light sweat contribute to the well-being of your brain.

Exercising can be fun when you track your progress and set and try to achieve goals. If you need some support, join a class or share your workout with a friend to help you stay on course. I find working with a personal trainer (if it is within your budget) is rewarding and enlightening. It is all about coordinating your body with your brain.

Not only will exercising boost your brain,
making it a habit will help you prolong your life.

Secret 61
Feed Your Brain

Your brain needs to be nourished to maintain your mental health in much the same way your body needs nutrients to keep physically fit. In order to concentrate, focus, and keep mentally alert throughout each day the brain must have a steady flow of energy. Not all foods supply the nutrition that gives your brain the boost it requires. It is important to be selective and certain that you are consuming brain foods in your daily diet. Among them are those that help prevent or lessen development of cognitive diseases.

Here are several foods recommended by nutritionists that will help you maintain a sharp, healthy brain.

Oily fish: Trout, mackerel, salmon, herring, sardines, pilchards, and kippers are good sources of omega-3 fats that are good for the healthy function of the brain.

Whole-grain products: Grains supply energy in the form of glucose to your brain. Choose brown cereals, granary breads, and brown pastas for yours.

Vitamins: B6, B12, and folic acid reduce homocysteine in the blood. Homocysteine increases risk of cognitive impairment.

Veggies: Leafy greens, asparagus, tomatoes, red peppers, and broccoli have qualities that enhance cognitive function and improve brain power.

Garlic: Garlic is high in the sulfur compound allicin and has over a dozen vitamins and a little of everything we need.

Berries: Blueberries and black currents are high in vitamin C and increase mental agility.

Pumpkin seeds: A handful a day is all you need for the supply of zinc that will enhance your memory and training skills.

Sage: Sage is known to improve memory. Even a dash now and then will help. There's more. Arabs, Chinese, and Gypsies believe sage is the key to a long life.

Nuts: Nuts are a great source of vitamin E, which helps prevent cognitive decline.

These foods are not only good for your brain and great for your overall well-being but you will enjoy their great taste. However, there are those that are harmful and should be avoided at all costs. Here are a few for your "not to eat list":

margarine	regular soda	beef hot dogs (try chicken or turkey)
whole milk	diet soda	deep dish pizza (eliminate sausage and
energy drinks	theatre popcorn	meat, try veggies)
processed foods	packaged sandwiches	
bagels	toaster pastries	

If you sense that your mind is a little foggy, sluggish, or slowing down, it's wise to check with your doctor or a qualified health-care professional who can suggest a regimen of helpful supplements.

Be sure to include brain foods in every meal
and avoid foods that are harmful.

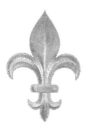

XIII. Face Your Sexuality Head On

Secret 62
(NUMBER)
Sexuality—For Women Only

Most of my Secrets have general benefits for all sexes and orientations—women, men, and the LGBT (lesbian, gay, , bisexual, and transgender) community. Since I am a straight woman, I discuss the issue of sexuality from that viewpoint. It is how I live, what I have experienced, and what I relate to. However, there are some points I make that have insight for those of any sexual orientation. So no matter what your gender or orientation, read on if you choose.

The world is changing rapidly, particularly in technology where new concepts pop up seemingly at every moment. Changes also reach beyond the technical, to our physical beings, our attitudes, and every aspect of our lives—including how we view and express our sexuality.

Since you have read at least some of my Secrets if not all, you are mature and more than likely over thirty. You have been there. You have experienced sex. According to fifty-three-year-old actress Kristin Todd Scott Thomas, "Experience is sexy." She should know. She is an English beauty, the paragon of cool, and star of Four Weddings and a Funeral and The English Patient.

As time has passed you may have begun to raise questions about the issue of sex and your own sexuality. What is sex at your age? What is sex at any age? As one grows older, does sexual desire diminish? If it does, are there ways to restore it? What does sex mean to you—how do you define sex? We each have our own definition based on our experience, dreams, and fantasies. Is it proper to fantasize or dwell on the subject of sex at any age? Are your feelings normal, acceptable? How much do you care? Do you care at all? Since you are reading this Secret, you care, even a little!

Dr. Gina Ogden, a family, marriage, and sex therapist offers comments about some common misgivings. She has authored several books with concepts that break away from old beliefs and unite sex with the body, mind, heart, and spirit. In her book The Heart and Soul of Sex, she sets forth encouraging tenets she labels Desiderata or "things you desire." These ten rights for women are designed to help you see your way through sexual dilemmas, help you overcome them and enjoy and add years to your life.

Desiderata: Your Right to Intimacy and Pleasure

1. I have a right to my own body and all of its sensations, including pleasure and pain.

2. I have a right to think my own thoughts, whatever they may be.

3. I have a right to feel the full range of my emotions—excitement, joy and anger, sorrow and depression, love and fear—whether or not my feeling them is acceptable to others.

4. I have a right to acknowledge my memories, whether they are memories of delight or abuse, and to base present relationship decisions on them.

5. I have a right to be—or not to be—a sexual person at all ages and stages of my life and a right to choose how I define what I mean by sexuality.

6. I have a right to expect my partner to respect my body, thoughts, feelings, and general well-being and a right to insist on respect.

7. I have a right to ask for what I want.

8. I have a right to say no to any sexual encounter that feels unsatisfying or threatening—physically, emotionally, spiritually, or sexually.

9. I have a right to say yes to pleasure that is physically, emotionally, spiritually, and sexually safe.

10. I have a right to feel good about saying yes or no to "things I desire."

Now that you may have accepted your rights to intimacy and pleasure you should be ready to experience both the physical and emotional complexities as well as the benefits of sexual encounters, which I discuss in the next Secret.

Secret 63

The Complexities and Benefits of Sex—For All

There have been myriad polls conducted to answer current questions on sex since the 1950s when the Kinsey Reports announced sexual behavior patterns to the world. One of the most recent, from the Institute of Sexuality and Intimacy at the Harvard Medical School, reports that from a strictly biological perspective, sex is "another hormone-driven bodily function designed to perpetuate the species."

The study reveals that sex is far more complex than the physical and encompasses a splendid panoply of emotions—tenderness, love, excitement, longing, anxiety, and disappointment. And as we mature (with some of us finding ourselves without partners) we question or reevaluate our sexuality.

The Harvard report defines sex as more than the so-called act of "genital-to-genital contact." There are pleasurable activities that involve other parts of the body—the mouth, the hands, the breasts, and sensitive areas of the skin—which when caressed can create erotic sensations.

You don't always need a partner to enjoy sex. Watching films, fantasizing, and masturbating are all acceptable methods of achieving gratification. However, if you run into a problem and need help, the specialists say there are always sex therapists in the wings to give you the self-assurance you seek.

Beyond these pleasurable intimacies, studies by British and other American researchers show there are physical benefits from the joy of sex. You may live longer, you use up to three hundred calories each time you indulge, your pelvic muscles along with your back, thighs, glutes, and abs are strengthened, and pain may be reduced. During orgasm the chemical oxytocin flows from the brain and appears to release endorphins—the body's natural painkillers—into your system. The medical profession says there are more and suggests you ignore the old-fashioned taboos and always practice safe sex.

So don't hesitate! Face your sexuality head on!
Indulge in the complexities and enjoy the benefits of sex.

XIV. Keeping Current

Secret 64
(NUMBER)

Curiosity Ensures a Happy, Healthy Mind
An Inquiring Mind Ensures a Happier, Healthier Life!

Curiosity may kill the cat, but for us humans an inquiring mind can add years to our lives. I have always been curious, and often my curiosity is so consuming that I am distracted from my work. Fortunately, most of the subjects that intrigue me relate to my work. Today, for example, I felt curious about curiosity, so I researched it. Among information I discovered is that an active sense of curiosity has countless benefits, most importantly its tendency to create happiness.

Happiness, according to an international study of more than ten thousand individuals, is viewed as more coveted than success, wealth, knowledge, maturity, relationships, wisdom, or the meaning of life. So if you are like most of the people in the world and seek happiness and a long life, build an inquiring mind and enjoy its benefits.

What are curiosity's benefits? What does it do for us?

Curiosity affects our memory positively
and stimulates the brain to enhance learning.

Curiosity is a powerful motivator. When your curiosity is stimulated, the brain becomes more active and you in turn become more motivated. You will be better, not only at learning your subject of interest, but also at learning unrelated information. In addition, curiosity increases activity in the hippocampus, a section of the brain that helps improve your memory.

How you can cultivate an inquiring mind

First: The best way to start is to be more aware of curiosity in your daily life.

Second: Take part in new and uncertain activities rather than focusing on the familiar. The familiar is comforting. The unfamiliar is exciting.

Third: Keep your mind open to building knowledge. Create a desire to learn more. Delve deeper into what you already know.

Page 78

Fourth: Seek the elements of surprise in typically boring everyday tasks. They are there. With an enlightened sense of curiosity, you'll uncover them.

Fifth: Approach tasks as a game. Challenge yourself to find new or different ways of approaching and accomplishing a task, enjoyable or boring.

It works. It works for me. Throughout my life I experience and live the concept of each of my Secrets. I'm inspired and curious to learn why they add years to my life. My research is exciting and gives me happiness, the greatest benefit of curiosity.

Enjoy the challenge. Increase your curiosity.

Secret 65
Toddlers to Teens Are Today's Tech Gurus
Ask your grandkids when you need help with your cell phone.

For us grown-ups, keeping pace with technological advancements can be a challenge. But not for kids. A friend's fourteen-year-old daughter showed me how to use my new smart phone. In return, I gave her a little to add to her savings for the car she hopes to buy. One day last week, while having dinner at a local restaurant, I observed a three-year-old boy standing next to his parents at a nearby table focusing on his smart phone while ignoring his hot, delectable meal. I have seen this happen often with both little girls and boys.

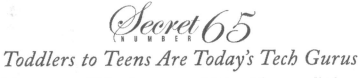

According to the 2013 *A Common Sense Research Study*, 75 percent of all youngsters up to age eight have access to at least one of the newer mobile devices. Since kids are the tech geeks of today, why not call on one in your family to help you with your device?

A newspaper in my county runs a full page of letters from grammar school students on a different subject every week. Recently the paper published the kids' epistles about their views on their parents' and grandparents' grasp of technology. Here are three revealing examples:

From Sawyer, grade 3: "My Mom does not understand Instagram. Instagram is an app. You can follow people, people can follow you, and you can like and post pictures on Instagram."

From Brody, grade 4: "The iPad is so popular these days, but I don't think so for next year. It seems odd to my grandparents and parents, and they said, "How do you turn it on?" They definitely do not get it because they haven't had this for a long time. And I've had it for nine years. They did not know how to turn it off or play a game or go on the Internet. I know how to do all these things."

From Gia, grade 4: "My grandparents do not understand electronics. They have no clue what they are doing. Almost every weekend they call my mom or dad to tell them what went wrong. The funny thing is they don't even want iPhones. They just want Droid. I think an iPhone would be too complicated for them."

The rest of the letters, about forty in all, are similar. They all show that kids are aware of their elders' inability to operate easy-to-use (for them) devices. Studies indicate that youngsters are frequent users of all digital media, including computers, handheld, and console video game players, cell phones, video iPods and iPad-style tablet devices. So don't hesitate to discuss your tech issues with them. *Good luck!*

Secret **66**

It's Never Too Late to Learn More

Engage in a reverse/reciprocal mentorship or consider going back to school!

I have a reverse mentorship with two members of the same family. I also have a third with someone who lives three thousand miles away. I didn't plan these mentorships. They evolved—because I have a passion for learning. For example, I have an exercise trainer, Jen. I benefit from her sessions, and she benefits from my Secrets. I asked her for someone to help with my cell phone and computer. Her fourteen-year-old daughter Emily (whom I have mentioned in other Secrets) has become my tech guru and learns from me as we work together. Through a friend I found an expert marketer in Arizona; he, too, learns from my Secrets.

It is never too late to learn!

First: Try to develop a reverse mentorship with someone in an age group different from yours: Millenials 18 - 34, Generation X, 35- 54, Baby Boomers, 55 - 69, Silent (but I'm not silent) 70 and older. Whether you mentor up or down, you will learn a lot either of both ways.

Next: Consider returning to school.

The reciprocal mentorship

With the world moving forward rapidly and with technology making new information available in seconds, it is critical to keep current and up to date. Developing a reciprocal mentorship with someone younger (or older) will help you move forward. If younger, seek out someone who will appreciate your experience and wisdom. Big companies like Burson-Marsteller, PricewaterhouseCoopers, and General Electric acknowledge the benefits of mentoring and encourage their employees to engage in the practice.

Returning to school

To keep current with advances in your industry or to prepare for a career change if your industry has become or is on the way to becoming obsolete, returning to school may be necessary, not an option. You can join the growing number of graduates and postgraduate students in their fifties and sixties who are choosing to take classes again.

Available financial help

Funding for school is not just for the young; it's available for those in the older groups as well. You can start by filling out a Free Application for Federal Student Aid (FAFSA). But make sure you are qualified. For most federal financial aid you must be enrolled at least half time in a degree or academic program. There are other opportunities, including tax breaks, 529 accounts, and scholarships designed specifically for mature students. You can try StudentScholarshipSearch.com and Fastweb.com for details.

It may take time to develop a reverse mentorship or to research classes designed to help you move on with your career. But it's worth taking advantage of the opportunities to learn. The effort can be a challenge but it may also be fun and rewarding and add years to your life.

XV. Loss Of A Loved One

Secret 67
N U M B E R

Grieve, Grieve A Lot, Then Move On

Most everyone has lost someone dear. Over the years, I have lost everyone in my family except my daughter Lisa. I am blessed to have her. I have grieved for those who have left me but am grateful to have had my husband Ralph help me through those sad times. Then he, too, was gone. As I grieved for him, I met Blair Pogue, the assistant pastor of the church I joined to seek solace. She commended me on my strength, strength I did not know I had. She suggested I share that strength with others in need. At the time, I wasn't ready. Not then. After several months had passed, I found that I was. I began to write the book I mention in several of my Secrets and on my Facebook page, *Move On: Reinvent Yourself, Find Contentment, I Did!* In this Secret I include a few brief comments from the book on "Ways to Handle Grief" and in the next Secret, "Enjoy New Life Options."

The shock and the grief

When you lose someone you love, you experience shock, fear, neglect, rejection, betrayal, guilt, anger, bewilderment, numbness, despair. Not every person will feel all of these, but everyone will experience a few with great intensity. You will feel and continue to feel many of these emotions until your inner strength returns and brings back your serenity.

> *"Sometimes we need to be alone with our grief and our memories. We just need to guard against making this our only response, for it's not healthy."*
> —Evangelist Billy Graham

You are entitled to grieve, grieve a lot. Cry, cry a lot. Talk, talk a lot. Talk with friends and family alike. Pour out your heart to them, for they want to be there for you. Grieve more. Grieve and cry as long as it takes. How long you grieve, experience other trying emotions, and go through the journey of renewal is different for everyone. There comes a time when we must all let go of our grief—the deep pain and hurt, while holding onto the healing memories. We must put the grieving behind us and move on. Always keep in mind Billy Graham's caveat that making grieving our only response is not healthy.

Letting go of grieving within a reasonable time
will help you take charge of your life.

My book *Move On: Reinvent Yourself, Find Contentment, I Did!* offers comprehensive information on finding contentment after losing a loved one.

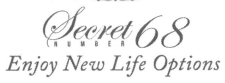

Secret 68
Enjoy New Life Options
Are you ready to embrace a new life?

Before you move on to undertake one or more of the new life options I list below, it is wise to have let go of much of your grief as discussed in Secret 67. You may have moved on, on your own, or found answers in my book Move On . . . I Did! No matter what helped you cross the bridge, or whether you are ready to begin a new life, you may want to review these options that will lead you to contentment.

Some New Life Options

A new significant other: When you have lost someone you love dearly, you may reject even the thought of a new relationship as I did when I lost my husband after a loving fifty-eight-year marriage. Many months later I unexpectedly entered a mutually caring friendship. Leo Tolstoy wrote, "To say that you love one person all your life is like saying a candle will burn all your life." Just be cautious! Make sure you select a trustworthy, compatible partner.

A new type of relationship: There is more than one type of socially and legally acceptable relationship in today's changing world. Any one (or two) may give you the life you wish. Not only has the world changed, you may have as well. You can select someone of the same sex; of a different race, religion, or culture; as a great friend or as a companion; as a confidant; as a live-in partner; or someone much older or much younger than you. It is your choice—whomever you feel comfortable with. Again, just be cautious.

Unconditional love: The emptiness and loneliness you experience when you have lost your love can be filled with the unconditional love of a pet. If you don't have or are allergic to the traditional dog or cat, there are many other loveable creatures that make great companions and will always requite your love. You will find a special critter that wants to be there for you. It can be love at first sight when you spot the one you didn't even know you were seeking. For more about unconditional love, see Secret 83.

A Dream Job: You've been grieving and out of touch with some aspects of your life, including your job. If the job you have is a dream job, return to it as soon as you can. If not, try to focus on finding a new one by following these steps: prepare a plan, determine a realistic schedule, network in person and on the Internet, attend job fairs and virtual job fairs, and be sure to follow up on your interviews. Always remember to spend more time off line than on line. Off line is where the jobs are!

Positive Pursuits with a Purpose: There is nothing more rewarding and satisfying than working on a project with a purpose for yourself or someone else or for a charity or fulfilling your civic duty as a political volunteer. As Mark Twain said, "The best way to cheer yourself up is try to cheer someone else up."

Pleasurable Pursuits: You owe yourself the joy of pleasurable pursuits. If you are still grieving, spend quiet time alone every day for an hour or two with a book or resting on a comfortable lounge listening to your favorite music. As time passes, move on to pursuits away from home, alone or with friends—at luncheons, dinners, a spa, sports events, and performances of the arts. When you are ready, pack your bags and travel to places you have always wanted to visit.

Your new life options are endless. These are just a few that show you that the world is full of wonders for you to enjoy. For more options you can check the Internet or get a copy of my book, *Move On . . . I Did!* from a library or Amazon.com. *Move On* includes long comprehensive chapters on each of the above options and much more.

XVI. Optimism

Secret 69
The Characteristics of an Optimist

Just recently, years after I coined my mantra "You must want to live a long life and view living with grace and acceptance," I came across the results of a study of five thousand individuals that reveals the strongest link to happiness and overall satisfaction in life. It is self-acceptance. Thinking positively, as an optimist, has scores of advantages, not the least of which is adding years to your life. The charity organization that conducted the research, Action for Happiness, released their findings, Ten Keys to Happier Living. They are listed here, spelling out the acronym Great Dream.

Giving: do things for others
Relating: connect with friends
Exercising: take care of your health
Appreciating: be aware of the world around you
Trying out: never stop learning

Direction: set reachable goals
Resilience: look for ways to bounce back
Emotions: be positive
Acceptance: be comfortable with who you are
Meaning: be part of something bigger than you

If you are an optimist, you already have most if not all of these attributes and live a happy life. If you are not and would like to be, practice one or more of the keys every day until they become a part of how you live. Then you will experience the amazing benefits of optimism, which I discuss in the next Secret.

Secret 70
The Benefits of Optimism and How to Beat the One Negative

Research has shown that optimists are healthier, happier, and more likely to live than pessimists to be centenarians. However, there are studies that reveal that optimists are unrealistic and unhinged from reality and have difficulty coping with unanticipated road blocks. The results prove that moderately happy people and pessimists, as negative thinkers, are prepared for obstacles and are more successful in finance, education, and politics.

To overcome the one negative of positive thinking, turn yourself around and become a Realistic Optimist. You will continue to hope for the best, be attuned to potential threats, and be able to handle adversities.

Optimists, whether unhinged or realistic (I happen to be realistic), have advantages far beyond pessimists, who view life negatively and have limited successes. Madeline Vann, MPH, Tulane University, New Orleans, a medical writer, lists some of the benefits optimists enjoy. They

- age more healthfully
- are able to improve relationships
- have better self-esteem
- make better decisions
- experience less stress and can better handle stress
- are more committed to goals
- are more likely to achieve goals
- are more satisfied with life
- have a strong sense of hope
- are more engaged and persistent in work
- make better athletes

If you are not an optimist and would like to become one, try some of these ways to help you enjoy the benefits of thinking positively. You can practice yoga, meditate, develop relationships with optimists, participate in spiritual or religious activities, and avoid negative thoughts and self-ridicule like "I'm an idiot" or "I was stupid."

Join the club of optimists and add years to your life!

Page 86

XVII. Delectable, Healthful Drinks

Secret Number 71

A Daily Glass of Red Wine
Will Add Years to Your Life*

The benefits of red wine, happily, are well documented. Here are six:

Benefit 1. You live longer than your friends who abstain. Studies have shown that drinking in moderation is good for the brain, helps preserve your memory, and protects against some forms of dementia. In fact, an article in *Neuropsychiatric Disease and Treatment* notes a test showing that moderate drinkers are 23 percent less likely to have memory problems than those who drink no alcohol.

I was drinking a glass of red wine every evening before I was aware of its long-life benefits. I drink just one glass a day. However, my birthday is coming up soon and I may celebrate with an extra goblet—just one more is still in moderation!

There are several more benefits,
which I support here with studies,
but there are caveats! (See the end of this Secret!)

Benefit 2. Studies show that wine is good for your heart. Could that be a reason why the French have one of the lowest heart attack rates in the world? According to Harvard University researchers, drinking moderate amounts of alcohol is one of eight proven ways to reduce the risk of coronary heart disease. Antioxidants in the skin and seeds of red grapes, called flavonoids, are credited with reducing the risk of heart disease.

Benefit 3. Red wine can uplift your mood, can be relaxing, and can lessen stress. Research from the HUNT Study in Norway revealed that moderate drinkers have a lower risk of depression than those who do not imbibe.

Benefit 4. Wine wards off some diseases. Research has revealed that resveratrol in the skin of red grapes may help those with diabetes regulate their blood sugar and lower blood glucose levels. Other studies indicate that moderately drinking men are less likely to be diagnosed with prostate cancer.

Benefit 5. Researchers in the United States and Spain report that red wine can prevent the common cold. The studies show that antioxidants are responsible.

Benefit 6. Contrary to popular opinion, an article in the Journal of Biological Chemistry by Purdue University researchers indicates that wine helps control your weight. Piceatannol, converted from resveratrol, "blocks insulin's ability to activate genes that carry out further stages of fat cell formation."

Now enjoy your dinnertime goblet of wine!

**The caveats: experts caution that
you will not reap the benefits of red wine if you overindulge
(more than two glasses a day for men and one for women)
and you must exercise regularly.*

Secret 72
White Wine Can Add Years to Your Life Too!

If you prefer white wine but feel obliged to switch to reap the health benefits of red, you no longer have to! Studies have proved white wine can also improve your health and extend your life. In fact, many leading researchers now believe that the neglected white is just as healthy as its darker cousin. Among them there are a few who admit they prefer the white, which may well have motivated them to study its benefits!

So what are those benefits?

The explanation lies in both the scientific and the technical.

Two of the foremost health experts, one at the University of Connecticut and the other at the University of Milan, found that white also has cardio-protective benefits that prevent heart attacks and other cardiac problems, while also protecting blood vessels and kidneys.

However, the benefits provided by white wines do not stem from the same compounds as those of reds. Red wine contains resveratrol, which gives it antiaging and heart-healthy properties, while white has the antioxidants tyrosol and hydroxytyorsol, which are also good for the heart. White wines, including champagne, may have even greater antioxidant properties than red.

Further, scientists have found that white wine activates sirtuin 1, the generic protein that helps to slow down the aging process. Their research also shows that white wine has many more advantages, including boosting your immune system, acting as an anti-viral agent, increasing the functioning of the brain, and raising good HDL cholesterol.

However, not all white wines offer these life-extending benefits. The best are those made from organic grapes grown and processed without chemicals and pesticides. Deborah Gavito, founder and wine director of the first organic bar in the United States—the Counter Vegetable Bistro and Organic Bar in New York City—recommends six organic or biodynamic whites that are palate pleasing and good for your heart.

Soave: A light and delicate white wine made from garganega grapes:
   Soave Classico, Corte Sant'Aida Vigne di Mezzane
   Inama Soave Classico

Torrontés: An aromatic Argentinean white that blends flavors of flowers and fruit:
   Yellow + Blue Torrontés
   Michel Torino Cuma Torrontés

Chardonnay: The best-known, most popular US white, buttery and bold, oaked or unoaked:
   Grgich Hills Chardonnay (Napa Valley)
   La Soufrandiere Pouilly-Vinzelles les Quarts (France)

There are several other European whites that have equal health advantages, mainly from Italy and Germany.

Now that you are ready to imbibe and enjoy the benefits of white, you must practice the caveats that are the same as for reds:
drink in moderation, no more than one goblet or glass a day,
and be sure you maintain your exercise regimen.

Secret 73

The Benefits of Green and Other Teas

I drink six or more cups of Green Tea every day!

I have been drinking green tea most of my adult life. Though Green Tea is the best known of the beneficial teas, the others worth trying are black, white, oolong, and rooibos. I just recently learned that Green Tea is the healthiest beverage on the planet!

Results of studies made with thousands of Japanese participants confirm and support the following list of benefits. Green tea is full of antioxidants and nutrients with powerful, positive effects for your body, brain, and overall well-being. However, it is wise to select the higher quality of green teas, since there are a few that contain high levels of fluoride. Nonetheless, lower qualities also have benefits.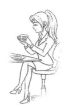

The benefits of green tea and select others*

Green Tea

• contains several bioactive compounds that improve your health, including polyphenols, such as flavonoids and catechins, which are powerful antioxidants, and epigallocatechin gallate (EGCG), which treats various diseases and also contains small amounts of minerals that are also good for your health.

• improves your physical performance by increasing fat burning and boosting your metabolic rate. The caffeine in tea (less than in coffee) mobilizes the fatty acids from the fat tissues and makes them available for use as energy.

• improves the functions of the brain. The limited amount of caffeine in green tea is enough to stimulate the brain to improve your mood, vigilance, reaction time, and memory without causing the "jittery" effects of too much caffeine. Green Tea also contains the amino acid L-theanine, which can cross the blood-brain barrier

• improves dental health. The catechins in green tea can inhibit the growth of bacteria and some viruses. This can lower the risk of infections, improve dental health, lower the risk of cavities, and reduce bad breath.

• reduces the risk of several diseases, including type #2 diabetes, cardiovascular disease, some cancers, Alzheimer's, and Parkinson's.

• helps you live a longer life!

*From the website Authority Nutrition.

*With all the benefits of green tea,
why would anyone choose to continue
to just drink coffee?*

Secret 74
The Magic of Smoothies
A Delectable, Healthful Drink

What we drink every day strongly impacts our health and how long we may live. We are constantly warned about the negatives of several types of soda, diet beverages, energy drinks, and overindulging in alcohol. Sure, milk, green tea, red and even white wine and chocolate drinks are all beverages that are good for you. But you can also always count on a smoothie! Not only can one glass quench your thirst or be a dessert or a full breakfast, but you can choose from dozens of healthful, delectable recipes that you can make yourself or enjoy at an eatery or buy in a food market.

Smoothies are a combination of ingredients you toss into a blender and presto, in five minutes, you have your smoothie. There are scores of ingredients to choose from to make the mixes; among them are fruit, milk, tofu, berries, nuts, spices, herbs, juices, yogurts, greens like kale and spinach, and ice. They can be topped off with seeds, chopped nuts, shredded coconut or tiny bits of fresh fruit.

Here's one to tempt your palate:

Kiwi Strawberry Smoothie
Ingredients for two servings
1 banana   6 strawberries
1 kiwi   1/2 cup vanilla frozen yogurt
3/4 cup pineapple and orange juice blend
Directions: *Place the juice blend in a blender. Dice the banana, kiwi, and strawberries and place them and the frozen yogurt in the blender. Blend until smooth.*
Try it, you'll love it.

In the next Secret you will find a few tips on how to make sure your smoothies are the best ever, along with one of my favorite recipes.

Enjoy the healthful benefits of a smoothie every day!

Secret 75
How to Make the Best Smoothies

It's almost impossible to make a smoothie that is not delectable. But to make sure that yours are the best possible, here are a few tips to help you create a winner each time you try:

- It is best to pour in the liquids as you begin, since it is easier on the blender.

- Start the blender at a low speed, then work up slowly to the higher speeds as the ingredients smooth.

- Consider using substitutes for dairy milk such as soy, hemp, rice, and almond. Try them and decide which you like best or alternate, since each has a unique flavor.

- Add texture to your smoothie by topping it off with seeds, finely chopped nuts, small squares of fresh fruit, or shredded coconut.

- For thick consistency, freeze the fruit you use and chop it to, again, conserve your blender.

• If you have made more of a smoothie than you can drink, pour the rest in an ice cube tray and blend it with the next one you make.

• Add the ice last and add as much as you choose. Three cubes are customary but add as many as you like for whatever creamy texture you want.

I offer two favorite smoothie recipes here that I make often, and you may choose to try:

Triple-Threat Fruit Smoothie
Ingredients, enough for four glasses

1/2 cup orange juice	*1 kiwi, sliced*
1 banana, peeled and sliced	*1/2 cup blueberries*
1 cup strawberries, diced	*1 (8 oz container) peach yogurt*

A Very Intense Fruit Smoothie
Rich, with a deep purple color
Ingredients, enough for two glasses
1 (10-ounce) package frozen mixed berries
1 (15-ounce) can sliced peaches or pears, drained
2 tablespoons honey
Directions: quick, easy and ready in three minutes.
Combine all the ingredients in a blender and mix until smooth.

There are some smoothies that are very rich, with extra thick consistencies. They often can serve as desserts and be poured into a bowl and enjoyed slowly with a spoon. (See the next Secret for Go Green with a Smoothie)

Experiment with all types of Smoothies
and be guided by these helpful tips.

Secret Number 76

Go Green With a Smoothie

A healthful smoothie is loaded with nutrients including proteins, vitamins, oil, fiber, and minerals that keep you healthy and extend your life. But you can count on green smoothies for a special nutritional-energy boost. They are particularly great for those who shun leafy veggies, since green smoothies offer an appealing way to get your daily dose of green. Greens are sky-high in nutrients. When they are mixed with fruit, yogurt, milk, and a healthy sweetener, the best of the flavors is enhanced. Include one or more of these greens in your smoothie and enjoy their benefits: kale, spinach, collards, watercress, beet greens, carrot tops, mustard greens, dandelion greens, chicory, along with others like honeydews and avocados.

You can start a daily regimen of smoothies with one of these or add another to your list:

A Green smoothie. rich and full of benefits

Pineapple Green Smoothie
Ingredients, enough for 1 1/2 cups
1/2 cup unsweetened almond milk   1 cup baby spinach
1/3 cup nonfat plain Greek yogurt   1/2 cup frozen pineapple chunks
1 cup frozen banana slices(about 1 medium)   1 tablespoon chia seeds
1–2 teaspoons pure maple syrup or honey (optional)
Directions: Pour the almond milk in a blender. Follow with the yogurt.

Then add the spinach, banana, pineapple, chia seeds, and a sweetener if you plan to use one. Blend the mixture until smooth. Sip it!

Another healthful green smoothie

Honeydew-Kiwifruit Smoothie
2 cups honeydew cubes   1 kiwifruit, peeled and diced
1 small Granny Smith apple, peeled, cored, and cut up
2–3 tablespoons sugar   1 tablespoon lemon juice   1 cup ice cubes
Honeydew and/or kiwifruit slices
Directions: Combine the honeydew, apple, kiwifruit, sugar, and lemon juice and place in a blender. Blend until smooth.
Add the ice cubes, and blend until the cubes are crushed and the mixture is slushy smooth. Top, if you wish, with the honeydew or kiwifruit slices.

You will find endless recipes for green smoothies on the Internet, but experiment and make your own. Create, have fun, and be sure to toss in a green and reap the benefits!

Secret Number 77
Enjoy the Benefits of Just One Cup of Coffee a Day

There was a time when I would enjoy three or four cups of steaming hot aromatic coffee every day. I loved its flavor so much that I would drink it black. Then, with the warnings about the harmful effects of high-caffeine beverages, I turned to decaf and then to green tea as my beverage of choice. Now, since the Italian longitudinal study of 1,445 individuals has shown that coffee has some awesome health benefits, I am reconsidering. The results indicate that drinking one to two cups a day (no more) significantly reduces the risk of MCI, mild cognitive impairment. In other words, coffee can improve your thinking process.

Because of the increase in coffee consumption over time to billions of cups a year, today's nutritionists have raised critical questions about the impact the stimulant has on the brain. They have concluded that "a steady stream of caffeine may be required for normal memory performance but increasing or decreasing consumption (from one cup a day) may result in impaired memory functioning."

There is another benefit to consider, particularly if you imbibe a few cocktails or shots of alcohol on a daily basis with friends at a bar or at home with your evening meal. The results of thirty-four studies of the amazing number of eight million men and women show that one cup of coffee a day may undo liver damage. However, to enjoy this benefit of restoring your liver, the process of that one daily cup of java must begin before you have any symptoms of the condition.

Therefore, if you want to ensure you protect your brain and your liver and you want to live a healthy, long life, don't indulge or overdo; limit your intake to just one cup of coffee a day.

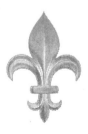

XVIII. Pursuits with a Purpose

Secret 78
(NUMBER)

The Rewards of a Pursuit With a Purpose

There is nothing more rewarding and gratifying than engaging in a pursuit that has a purpose—for yourself, for someone else, for a charity, or for all three. Undertakings like these add joy and years to your life. Best-selling author and cofounder of the Chopra Center for Wellness, Deepak Chopra, has this to offer on the subject of pursuing a purpose:

> *"Purpose gives you fulfillment and joy*
> *and can bring you the experience of happiness."*

A personal pursuit: Finding and pursing one's own purpose can be more challenging than undertaking a pursuit to help others. You must encompass the critical task of how you view, handle, and carry out your life's work—your career—and how you relate to family. This task is bigger than self and takes time for introspection. You are fortunate if you are already on your path. If not, you may consider these concepts:

- What are your talents?
- What are your strengths?
- What are you drawn to—what do you enjoy?
- What are your passions?

Make a list for each of the questions. Eliminate all your answers but the most important one in each category. Review your list. Discuss them with people who are close to you and whom you trust. Take time to contemplate your answers. Weigh the talks you had with your friends. Determine your purpose. Pursue it!

Having purpose in your chosen field of endeavor adds meaning to your life and may contribute to a broader social benefit, to the greater good, and to a wider, global cause. With the rapid technological changes in our world, you may have to alter your purpose as time passes. Be alert to when that comes. Change or adjust your purpose and continue to enjoy fulfillment. I feel blessed to have found mine—to help others live a happy, healthy, long life, as I do.

> *In the next Secret, I offer pursuits with a purpose*
> *you may undertake for someone else and for multitudes.*

Secret 79

The Importance of a Purpose In Retirement

My Secrets are positive revelations on how to live a full, happy, long life as I do. I avoid the negative. However, in a recent issue of AARP: The Magazine, there is a powerful message supporting the importance of having a purpose in life:

> "Men more than women define themselves by their careers. At retirement, they can lose self-worth which can lead to depression, excessive drinking and other health problems. Studies show that having a higher purpose in life significantly reduces the risk of death among older adults and can even slow or prevent cognitive decline."

This statement speaks eloquently about pursuing a worthwhile purpose if you choose to have a happy, long life.

In Secret 78, I discuss the challenges, the rewards, and the significance of having a personal purpose. In this Secret I suggest pursuits in which you can engage, first, to help individuals and, second, to reach out to help others through one or more of the multitude of charities. These are meant to and can prepare you to move on to establish a purpose of your own design.

Pursuits with a purpose to help someone else: You won't have to go far to find a friend, a relative, or a neighbor who will fulfill your purpose of helping others. When I was writing *Move On: Reinvent Yourself, Find Contentment, I Did!* I had just completed the second chapter, "The First Hurdle: The Shock and the Grief," when one of my neighbors lost her husband to Alzheimer's. I offered her a copy. After she read it she told me, "What you have written helps me handle my grief. Your words are comforting and give me peace." She confirmed that I was fulfilling my purpose.

You can fulfill yours by driving someone home-bound in need to the doctor, to church, or to shop or arrange for an expert to repair an appliance or tutor a child in a subject you know. The ways you can help and render your purpose are endless.

Pursuits with a purpose that help multitudes: A positive pursuit in the broadest sense reaches out to more people than any other. This pursuit is volunteerism. You do not need a special talent to be a volunteer.

There are assignments on every level from filing and answering the phone to organizing a fund-raiser and giving a speech on behalf of the organization. The causes are overwhelming in number. Among them are literacy, children's welfare, food kitchens, religious charities, conservation, medical research, adoption agencies, wildlife preservation, animal charities, housing for the poor, the arts, helping veterans, and many more.

When you practice a pursuit with a purpose, you give help and pleasure. According to statesman, publisher, inventor Benjamin Franklin:

"Whoever pleasure gives, shall joy receive."

Be passionate about your purpose, receive joy, and add years to your life!

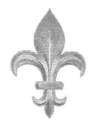

XIX. Fun Exercises

Secret 80

Dancing Has More Benefits Than Running

Want a respite from your exercise regimen without losing its benefits? Try dancing. Believe it or not, there are hundreds of types of dance you can choose from. Many have more benefits than standard exercise. And most have a special plus that you don't find in many exercise programs. Since you dance with a partner, not only is dancing fun and pleasurable—if it someone with whom you have a relationship—you will feel closer and your bond will be strengthened.

But my Secrets are not just about pleasure, but about health benefits that contribute to your living a long life. Here are some that dancing offers:

Balance: Many dance moves require hesitating on one foot and holding positions for moments that call on your balance. These practices build up strength in stabilizing muscles and your core and help maintain overall balance.

Muscle tone: The fast pace, continuous exertion, and occasional unusual positions in balance provide muscles with resistance. These develop strength and muscle tone in your legs and fanny and flatten your tummy.

Flexibility: Dancing increases the flexibility of your body. Most dance lessons include warm-up sessions that consist of a lot of stretching.

Posture: To be a good dancer you must think of your posture: roll your shoulders back and lift up your chin and chest. Remembering to do these can carry over to improving your natural posture.

Burning calories: Some dances increase circulation, improve stamina, and burn as many as five to ten calories a minute—a fun way to lose some weight if that is what you want.

Studies have found several more benefits for dance, including the improvement of your memory, your mood, and your kinesthetic awareness. Further, dance raises HDL (good cholesterol), lowers LDL (bad cholesterol), increases metabolism more than running, and adds to lung capacity.

I don't suggest you abandon your exercise program, but on occasion find time to enjoy the benefits of dance.

Secret Number 81

Experience the Élan of Fencing

All my life, I have been fascinated by the lure of fencing. It all began with watching the skillful moves of Errol Flynn in long-ago films and studying medieval history—when swords were the weapons of choice and duelers fought to the death. Fencing, based on centuries of tradition, is elegant, graceful, and prestigious. Today, it is a modern combative sport, a challenge both physically and tactically between two opponents—an effective blend of patience, discipline, and determination. No longer a duel of survival, fencing is a challenge of wits.

I had always hoped to engage in the sport, and finally, when I was in my early seventies, I began. It was a thrilling experience, but one I had to forgo when my husband fell victim to Parkinson's disease. However, I now plan, once again, to take up my swords and gear and reengage in my sport of choice.

Fencing goes beyond being a sport; it is an art, a body booster that is more of a challenge than most other exercise regimens. A fencing session is a full-body workout that places physical fitness demands on muscles from the feet and lower legs all the way up to the shoulders, arms, and neck. Fencing challenges and improves the body's performance, and research shows that the sport has proven health and fitness benefits.

Among them, fencing

- improves balance and timing
- provides a fun way to get fit and stay in shape
- increases focus and concentration
- boosts mental strength
- increases the nimbleness of hands and feet
- improves speed, agility, flexibility, and reflexes
- hones strategic thinking and decision-making skills
- offers a dynamic circle of peers and mentors (friends)
- can add years to your life

I hope I have sufficiently intrigued you to consider pursuing this art. I suggest you check the Internet, bookstores, and/or libraries to learn more about the grace, elegance, and fascination of fencing. I assure you, you will be challenged and excited, whether you choose to take lessons or just learn more about this centuries-young sport.

XX. Other

Secret NUMBER 82

Performing in Today's IT World

The day before I planned to work on this Secret, I experienced a near-panic IT (information technology) pressure situation. When I returned home after a rewarding morning interview I participated in about my next book, I was greeted with an urgent voice-mail.The message was about a letter I had drafted that had to be e-mailed by four that afternoon to the board of directors of a charitable organization for which I volunteer. I had to edit the correspondence, get approval from committee members, then e-mail it to six officers of the board. At two o'clock, my computer froze! I spent an hour trying to unfreeze it without success. Finally, I called a friend for help. I reached her but she was on a tight schedule and could spare only a few minutes. She tried to guide me by phone. Nothing worked. Sensing the urgency to get the letter out, and despite her own pressing matters, she said she would come to my home to try—a twenty-minute drive. She did. With difficulty, Jen solved my problem. The e-mail was sent at 3:55 p.m.

IT pressures are common occurrences, inevitable in today's world. When they are not solved quickly they can impact your health, cause stress, and often take years off your life. In several earlier Secrets, I address the management of stress caused by personal crises including divorce, financial problems, loss of a loved one, and other similar issues. Here, I offer ways to handle stress due to pressures in the workplace that help reach positive resolutions and achieve goals. Some are results of studies. Others are mine.

Be positive: Approach what you face as a challenge. Accept it as an opportunity that will add to your list of career accomplishments.

Do not react preemptively: Take a deep breath and proceed slowly with a clear mind.

Be realistic: Analyze and pinpoint the challenge. Determine how critical it is. Are there any deadlines? If so, what are they? What are the obstacles you may face?

Prepare for the encounter: Have a plan. Create a list of steps that you must undertake. Do them!

Focus on the task, not the outcome. Concentrate on your plan. Avoid concerns about winning or losing. They distract from your preparation and cause stress and anxiety.

Determine the worst that can happen: Anticipate the unexpected. What if there are more on their team than yours. What if the deadline is sooner than previously announced? What if . . . ? What if . . . ? Don't panic. Be ready to brace yourself, maintain your composure, and perform in the best way you can.

How did you successfully handle previous challenges? Reviewing your past successes will reaffirm your confidence and can produce another win. If you did it before you will do it again.

Share the pressure you have with a friend or coworker you trust. Studies have shown that talking about the pressure you feel lessens the stress and anxiety. You will be able to openly examine your feelings, view them more realistically and learn other ways to face and beat the challenge.

In my current situation, I didn't have time to act on all of these steps. However, having lived through many challenges, I took a deep breath and let as many as time permitted come into play. I won. I also had some help!

Good luck with your challenging encounters!

Secret 83

NUMBER

Enjoy Unconditional Love

The unconditional love of a pet will add years to your life.

If you already have a pet, no doubt you enjoy companionship and unconditional love. A family critter is fine, but one of your very own is even better. Poet and naturalist Henry David Thoreau once wrote:

"It often happens that one is more humanely related to a cat or a dog than to any human being."

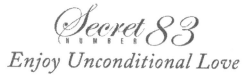

You don't have to welcome a dog or cat into your life, particularly if you are allergic to fur. There are scores of others animals and breeds to choose from. Nonetheless, I chose Niqui, my gentle whippet, who joins me for my daily morning walks. She also follows me wherever I go in my home, never barks, but does talk excitedly in her own special voice when I am about to feed her or give her a treat. Surprisingly she also talks with her ears in a language I have come to understand. I have unconditional love! (FYI: Her full name is Dominique, La Princesse de Poitiers.)

If, on the other hand, you choose a feathered friend, one of the exotics, or another small four-legged animal that is not very tame, you may be equally blessed. A former neighbor who just bought a farm told me his latest pet is a huge rabbit that hopped onto his porch and moved into his house and his heart.

You don't have a pet? Never had one? Give it a try! Visit a rescue kennel or a ranch that harbors all sorts of animals—you may find love at first sight and live happily -- and long -- ever after. Check the Internet for sources or the chapter on pets in my book *Move On! Reinvent Yourself, Find Contentment, I Did!* which includes helpful information and fun details like American presidential pets. Did you know that Theodore Roosevelt had a menagerie of twenty, among them a badger, a rat, a garter snake, and a one-legged rooster? That Calvin Coolidge had sixteen, including two raccoons, an antelope, and a pygmy hippopotamus?

There's more. Enjoy your search! You will find unconditional love!

Secret 84

Live Your Passing Years Raucously

Face your fleeting years
with enthusiasm, passion, courage, and raucousness.

Enjoy your maturing years with good humor and brandish your cane if you need one. I have to admit I did not include raucousness in my Secrets early on, but why not now? With caution and among friends, being boisterous and disorderly (the dictionary definition) can be inspiring and exciting. So, from Regina Barreca, professor of English at the University of Connecticut, I'm borrowing the act of raucousness and adopting it as one of my own.

Enthusiasm, passion, and courage have always been among my priorities for living a happy, healthy, sexy life. I welcome Regina's added spin on senior years by placing emphasis on what I consider sexy.

Fifty-seven-year-young Barreca has dispensed with the phrase "growing old graciously." As she has aged, she has changed her goal from "becoming contemplative and introspective" to "be more disruptive, seditious and boisterous." Also, along with brandishing a cane, since she might have to since her family has a history of bad knees, she will carry a flask. Whether it contains gin or Ensure, she declares she doesn't care. She simply wants to be able to "whip out a flask" without notice.

This upbeat professor, editor, and author of seven books offers you an alternative—she chooses to grow old not gracefully but gaudily. It just may add years to your life.

Secret NUMBER 85
The Three Elements of Existence
Unite the three elements of your being and add years to your life!

You will be secure and in control when you connect your spirit, your mind, and your body. Your spirit is the force that will guide you as long as you permit it to play an important role in your life. Your spirit helps your mind interact with your body and carry out your goals—improving your physical strength, maintaining your bodily fitness, and eliminating causes of stress. When you operate from an understanding of the interconnected nature of mind, body, and spirit, you will better understand the need and how best to exercise, relax, and meditate.

Just recently I learned how to manipulate my body (my muscles, my limbs, my neck, my back, all of it) to execute more efficiently and effectively the exercises my trainer Jen dictates. Before, I had done them by rote—simply reacting to command. However, when I mentally engage my body and focus on the moves I must make, something unique and exciting occurs. I feel in command. There is a deliberate connection—my mind and my body are united.

If you have trouble evoking your spirit or are not inclined to do so, you may prefer to call on your vital force—which may mean to you desire, control, or will power—to drive you to add years to your life. I prefer to rely on my spirit—which is far more knowing and aware than I.

Whatever or whoever helps you,
connect your mind with your body, be grateful, and accept!

Secret 86
Procrastination Can Help You Enjoy Life
Putting off tasks will help you enjoy and prolong your life!

Most of us consider the concept of procrastinating as a negative. I certainly did, and I never expected to include it as one of my Secrets. It's not a positive attribute, I kept telling myself, and I was about to remove it from my list. Yet the idea was deep in my psyche and would not let go. I decided to entertain myself and do some research to learn why it stayed with me. It took a lot of time, but eventually I was convinced. Why? Because I am a procrastinator by nature and so are a lot of very bright mature professionals, including artists, authors, scientists, technocrats and scores of others.

How does being a procrastinator prolong your life? Here are some reasons how and why!

First: Procrastinators are planners and doers.

Second: Many procrastinators make lists and we change them often.

Third: We have important projects that we put on the top of the list.

Fourth: We place household chores, running errands, and related tasks lower on the list and consider them unimportant.

Fifth: We feel, however, that we must take care of the lesser chores, which are easy and quick to complete to get them out of the way first. But we feel guilty for doing them because we are putting off the important project that may be the one that pays our bills.

Finally: By getting all the easy chores out of the way (procrastinating) we have delayed starting the most pressing project but no longer have a choice but to start it.

The secret is to become a productive procrastinator!

Here are a few tips on how:

1. Set aside an hour or two (or more) every day to concentrate on your important project.

2.Learn how to say no to requests that do not relate to that project.

3.Avoid interruptions and distractions.

4.Take your time. Work up slowly onto the core of your project.

5.Don't sweat the lesser projects; get on to the important one(s).

6.Prioritize your list and adjust it when necessary.

7.Outline your major tasks. Then break them down into small parts that can be taken on one at a time.

8.Plan a reward for yourself after each is completed: a ten-minute nap, a cup of coffee, a glass of wine, or a walk in the park. Or grab dinner with friends at your favorite restaurant.

9.Tell someone about what you are doing and when you will complete a part of or your entire project. The public commitment will help keep you on course.

You don't have to do all the above, just enough to make you a productive procrastinator! You will be pleased that you have completed your major projects and you will enjoy and add years to your life.

Secret 87

Telomeres: A Key to Aging Well

As I research background material for my Secrets, to support what I have practiced instinctively all my life, I am always inspired when I discover something unexpected. Telomeres is among the most fascinating of my discoveries. Dr. Richard Cawthon and fellow genetics researchers at the University of Utah suggest that if all the processes of aging could be eliminated and oxidative stress damage were repaired, they foresee that "people could live a thousand years."

An article from the University of Utah's Learn Genetics website provides a fascinating look:

Inside the nucleus of a cell, our genes are arranged along twisted, doubled molecules of DNA called chromosomes. At the ends of the chromosomes are stretches of DNA called telomeres, which protect our genetic data, make it possible for cells to divide, and hold some secrets to how we age and get cancer.

Telomeres have been compared with the plastic tips on shoelaces, because they keep chromosomes ends from fraying and sticking to each other, which would destroy or scramble an organism's genetic information.

Yet, each time a cell divides, the telomeres get shorter. When they get too short, the cells can no longer divide; it becomes inactive or "senescent" or it dies. This shortening process is associated with aging, cancer, and a higher risk of death. So telomeres also have been compared with a bomb fuse.

The article continues in great scientific detail. A quick summary shows that as an enzyme, telomerase, which remains active in human sperm and eggs that are passed down from one generation to the next, helps maintain the length of telomeres.

Researchers indicate the "if we used telomeres to 'immortalize' human cells, we may be able to mass produce cells for transplantation" to cure several debilitating diseases.

The human lifespan has increased considerably from the 1600s, when the average was thirty years. By 2012, the average life expectancy in the United States was seventy-nine. Some scientists predict the average life expectancy will continue to increase but many doubt it will ever be much higher than ninety.

*If you have become as fascinated as I with the subject
of telomeres and why they are the key to aging,
check the Internet to learn more.*

Secret 88

The Importance of Taking Care of Your Skin

Taking care of your skin may not lengthen your life but it will certainly keep you from looking your age. The sooner you begin a skin-care regimen, the more you are assured of maintaining a youthful glow and avoiding deep lines and wrinkles. It was when I turned eighty that my friends began to comment on the smooth state of my skin, and even now in my nineties I hardly have a visible dent. Recently during a visit to a dermatologist for a nail problem she solved for me, she asked what I used to wash my face. Just water, I told her, and then I apply a rich, thick lotion I have used for as long as I can remember.

Ways to care for your skin

Eat a healthy diet: Healthy food not only makes you feel good; it gives your skin a special texture and glow.

Make sure your diet includes vegetables, fruits, whole grains, lean proteins, and vitamins—and stay clear of unhealthy fats and processed or refined carbohydrates.

Be gentle with your skin: Limit your bath or shower time, use warm, not hot water, avoid strong soaps, pat or blot your skin dry, and use an appropriate moisturizer.

Protect your skin from the sun: Fresh air and the out of doors are important for healthy skin, so take your regular walk in nature. But stay in the shade, use sunscreen, and wear protective clothing.

Control stress: Your state of mind and your emotions directly affect the condition of your skin. Focus on managing your stress as I suggest in earlier Secrets: practice yoga or check chapter 7 in my book, Move on . . . I Did!

Simply, live a healthy lifestyle! And check with your health-care provider or a dermatologist for the lotions best for the skin types of your face and other parts of your body. I attribute my smooth, healthy skin to my lifestyle—the positive way I view life. I also smile as often as possible to keep my face from drooping! It keeps me happy, and I go on like the Energizer Bunny.

Secret 89
Accept Offers of Love and Help

Most of us at some time in our lives are faced with one or more problems beyond our ability to solve alone. The situation is particularly challenging for those of us with a strong sense of independence who are reluctant to reach out for help. We, the strong, the independents, regretfully believe that accepting assistance is out of character with our spirit, our ability to cope, and a sign of weakness. Occasionally, we consider ourselves failures unless we solve our problems ourselves. It is imperative to remember this:

Those notions are far from the truth.

As human beings we are social animals. In order to achieve happiness and live rewarding long lives, we must interact and socialize with one another. If you are rejecting offers of help and would like to be more accepting, a good way to start is to understand why you shun help.

You may feel you will lose your independence. You may be rejected or considered a failure. You may show signs of inferiority or incompetence. You won't.

The next step is to realize that seeking help is not a weakness:

The media portrays heroes and leaders as independent and impervious to problems. Not so: they have many supporters and helpers to call on. Comparing yourself to others you consider successful and able to handle problems alone is unrealistic. Call on others as leaders do. Then accept the help with grace and gratitude.

Ask yourself if seeking help has benefits for you and/or the giver:

Separating yourself from others leads to isolation. Think of reciprocity. You, no doubt, have helped others. You can offer to trade expertise, skills, and advice. You will gain access to methods and ideas in your own field (or life) and share yours with others. You not only help yourself, you give strength to the giver. You both benefit.

Learn how to let others help you in ways you are comfortable:

Be cautious as to whom you reach out for help. Don't ask just anyone. Choose wisely and carefully. Avoid someone who will belittle you. Select someone you trust. Plan what you will say and go slowly in requesting your need.

Finally, prioritize your problems and view seeking help as sharing:

As you go about seeking help or advice, don't be apologetic, to yourself or to the person you ask. Prioritize your problems. Some you will find you can handle yourself and you may just need more information from others to solve alone. Only then, go the next step. Reach out to someone you trust, and be ready to offer your expertise in return. Swap your skills.

Problem solving can be a rewarding challenge
and you can reap the joys of sharing.

Secret 90
NUMBER

Don't Take Growing Old Sitting Down

A physical exercise regimen is touted as a promise not only to lengthen the life of your body but also to preserve your memory and boost your *brain power!* Of course! However, there is a caveat: In this computer age, there is a looming health risk that you will experience even if you exercise regularly. Put simply, *sitting is the new smoking.*

Spending fifteen minutes to a half hour of rugged exercise at the gym does not guarantee you will enjoy a healthy, long life if you spend the rest or a part of your work day hunched over your computer without taking a break. There have been several studies on sedentariness that have proved that prolonged periods of seated inactivity lead to diseases that take a toll on your health and shorten your life.

In other words, be aware of and respond to the adage "Move it or lose it!"

There are ways to avoid the sitting disease—methods that you should add to your regular physical activity, not replace it. These are easily performed whether you work at an office or at home. Dr. John Buckley, professor of applied exercise science at the University of Chester in England, suggests avoiding sitting for more than a half hour at a time. Here are a few ways to "move it" without disrupting your work.

Standing: Take a quick thirty-second to two-minute break standing up every half hour. Try standing on one foot briefly and then the other. Standing burns twice as many calories as sitting. You can alternate still sitting by swinging your legs back and forth to improve blood flow and prevent muscles and limbs from getting rigid.

Spurts of activity: Develop habits of walking such as to another room to the printer or copier; walk the stairs instead of taking the elevator; when you need to confer with a coworker, walk the corridor or hallway as you talk; and take coffee breaks and lunch walks rather than sit your desk.

Exercise Equipment:: Many employers are responding to the threat of the sitting disease and offer workers active sitting options that include ball chairs, cycling seats, the Locus desk, and the TrekDesk among others, as well as workstation floor mats. If you work at home, you can find workstations that are available at a variety of price levels.

The threat of the sitting disease goes beyond the workplace to lounging for hours at home watching television or sitting long periods in the theater, at a sports event, at a concert, or even for hours in traffic. Try to make a practice of planning to "move it" before each prolonged sitting session you may encounter.

Secret 9 1
NUMBER

Take Charge of Your Finances
Build a nest egg and secure peace of mind.

If you haven't started saving yet, start today. You will ensure living a happy, healthy, long life only if you build a nest egg that will give you peace of mind. Don't be hypnotized by the notion that you must save a certain amount of money or that you've waited too long to make a difference. Simply begin now. I began when I was thirteen with twenty-five cents of the three dollars I was paid in my first job (at ten cents an hour). It wasn't much but it was a beginning. I continued to put away some of what I earned each time I was paid and more when I could. Over the years, I have built a substantial nest egg—far less than the one-percenters, but enough so that I am quite comfortable and I can indulge in a few luxuries.

When I began my Secrets I hadn't planned to include one on finance, since I suggest you work with a financial adviser—and I still recommend you do. However, I was prompted to change my mind and offer a few tips in this Secret for those who need help in building a nest egg. My change of heart came when I met Steve (not his real name), who as a computer program designer in his late thirties was struggling to support his lovely wife and four little ones—three, five, seven, and nine.

When I happened to mention my financial comfort zone and how I achieved it, Steve, for the first time in his life, set out to regularly put aside some of his modest income. As a Hollywood stunt man during his twenties he had made millions and squandered every penny. He had sustained serious injuries (once he was in a coma for three months) and decided to leave the glamorous world of celebrity and, as a fan of my Secrets, live a long life. He says my advice has put him back on the right track.

This is a true story . . . as all of mine are!

This Secret is not about investment strategies. It is an introduction to how to attain and maintain financial security when you are read y to invest.

Decide now to build your nest egg.
You will achieve financial security, peace of mind and a long life.

First and foremost: If you have not yet started to save, don't delay. Start today!

Second: Establish realistic financial goals.

Third: Have a plan. Organize your income, your expenses, your savings with your assets and liabilities in such a way that that you will be able to meet your objectives.

Fourth: Create an emergency fund that will cover at least three months of expenses.

Fifth: Regularly check the status of your plan.

These steps are designed to get you started on your road to financial security. For more information and helpful financial forms for your plan you may reference chapter 11 of my book *Move On: Reinvent Yourself, Find Contentment, I Did!* To ensure success, I suggest you pursue the steps in depth by checking the Internet and/or books in libraries and bookstores.

Financial security is a major element in living a long life.

Secret NUMBER 92

Dare To Be Daring With a Touch of Whimsy In Your Day

I was inspired to write this Secret by a surprising remark from a friend in my exercise class as we were changing clothes in the women's locker room. "Oh," she exclaimed when she spotted my leopard-patterned panties, "that's fun. I will have to get some!" That was a lift for me for making someone happy and set me on to think of other ways to add touches of whimsy to our days.

For a start, there are scores of lingerie designs to give you a chuckle, including kittens, puppies, butterflies, flowers, and hearts, as well as brilliant colors, stripes, and geometric patterns. These fantasy fancies are not confined to women's fashions, as designers have not neglected men. They have come up with some daring masculine styles. You can be creative and daring on your own by wearing those T-shirts with crazy slogans and odd baseball hats, or dye your hair purple or orange—and how about a temporary, whimsical tattoo on your arm, ankle, or a place of your choice?

There are ways you can indulge in flights of whimsy that go beyond the obvious and personal. Think of the joy you feel when you hear the laughter of children or watch them at play. Join them. Spend an hour or two with your grandchildren, or if you don't have any, seek out your nieces and nephews or your neighbors' kids. Take them to a carnival, a circus, a horse show, a parade, an ice cream shop. Play ball with them in a park or take them Halloween trick-or-treating. You will share their laughter, get a big shot of whimsy, and earn the gratitude of their parents for giving them some extra quiet time away from their kids.

There is more than whimsy to enjoy when you spend time with little ones. You will be amazed and uplifted. According to a preschool teacher who works in the suburbs of Melbourne, Australia,

> "Children come to us with many strengths, competencies and capabilities. There seems to be no limit to their imagination, creativity, curiosity and inquiry. They are typically 'learning optimists.'"

Kids aren't for you? Try sharing some whimsical time with a friend or two or more. The more the merrier. Consider an old-fashioned escapade, a picnic in the country under a huge oak tree, blankets to rest on, loads of food and sparkling champagne to add extra sparkle. In winter, bundle up and trudge through heavy falling snow. Or hire a horse-drawn sleigh, and ride to the jingle of the sleigh bells. Sing along with songs you love and stop at your favorite pub for a hot toddy. End your day with a great night's sleep and dreams of the delights of whimsy.

Not only is there joy in wearing something fanciful or in spending a special time with kids or friends, you will find delight in the caprice of whipping up a new notion, especially when you gather with friends in your home or theirs to plan the next whimsical event.

Enjoy a lighthearted whimsy as often as you can
and add years to your life.

Secret 93

The Benefits of Keeping a Journal

One of the most important daily tasks I have engaged in for more than fifty years is writing in my journal. Another is making to-do lists. Both keep me organized, up to date, and on course. They are the last things I do before going to bed. I sleep soundly, for I know where I have been during the day (a necessary reminder that shows me what I have accomplished) and I am ready to start fresh when I get up the next morning.

There is one problem, however. I'm running out of space to store my steadily growing
number of journals!

After I began to keep a journal, I learned that there are many powerful and influential individuals today and in history who do or have done the same. The benefits go far beyond record keeping and being organized. The concept may be compared to taking on any new regimen such as exercising, which can also improve your diet and help you feel less stressed and be more patient. Journaling, too, can become a habit that has many benefits and can shape your life. It has done that for me.

Enjoy the power of the benefits!

Journaling

- serves as a springboard for your workday
- supports your ability to carry out your goals
- challenges your creativity
- clears your mind
- helps you handle your emotions
- improves ability to retain information and increase brain power and memory
- makes you a better and more facile writer
- keeps a record of your life

Over time you will find that keeping a daily journal helps you become more productive—the person you have always hoped to be—and create the life you have always wanted to live. You will be happier and healthier and add years to your life.

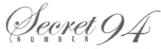

Secret Number 94

Move Slowly When You Make a Change in Your Life

There are times in our lives when we are faced with major changes that must be made. Perhaps you have lost someone through death, divorce, or betrayal; you've been fired or you are unhappy with your job, your boss, or your workplace environment; you need a new home; the pastor of your church has moved on and you are not pleased with the replacement; you may want to explore a new religion. The reasons are endless and may be as simple as seeking a new doctor, dentist, financial advisor, or even a new hairdresser or barber to replace the one with whom you have been content who has retired.

Changes are filled with challenges and unknowns
and are best approached slowly and with caution!

It is wise to pursue your change gradually to ensure that your transition is smooth, that your choice is right for you, and that your move is successful. Your decisions should be made from a place of strength, not from panic. This helps you add years to your life.

A place to begin, if you have not already done so, is to establish your identity and self-confidence as discussed in Secret 3 and follow the suggestions on setting goals in category III, "Lifetime Goals." Then, as you launch the steps in your change process, be guided by this quotation from William Shakespeare:

"Be patient as a gentle stream!"

First: Prepare a list of changes you want to make. Select two or three possible choices, then eliminate all but one. Take time to make sure you have made the right choice. Be ready for disappointments and to substitute another choice.

Second: Analyze the reasons why you made this choice: to increase your income, to have a more challenging job, a new living environment, just to get away for a while, to make new friends.

Third: Develop an inventory of what you have to offer and what you will need to ensure success. List your interests, your likes, dislikes, motivations, talents, and all your qualities that support your choice.

Fourth: Write a plan, akin to a business plan. Include your purpose, your goals, your resources, your finances, and the professional help you will need: an attorney, an accountant, and any others.

Fifth: Set a realistic timetable. Launch your change. Again, be patient.

> *"Whatever you can do or dream you can, begin it.*
> *Boldness has genius, power and magic in it."*
>
> Johann Wolfgang von Goethe

If you would like more information on these steps to help you move on, you may refer to chapter 5 in my book *Move On: Reinvent Yourself, Find Contentment, I Did!*

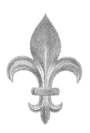

XXI. Love Every Year of Your Life

Secret 95
(NUMBER)

Build a Trove of Treasures: My Secrets to Happiness

As you celebrate each birthday, you launch upon new exciting adventures. What joy does your next year have in store for you? What new challenges await? What new trials will you overcome that will prepare you for the next? The wonders of the world outweigh and help us handle the difficult times and tragedies we each experience in our lives. We do become better as time passes—it will happen if you will it to!

These treasures give you great joys and add years to your life—but always keep this mantra in mind:

*You must **want** to live a long life*
and view living with grace and acceptance!

You need not practice all ninety-five Secrets, but here are a few suggestions to help you stay on track:

First: Make sure you have all the basics in category I in your regimen.

Second: Check through the rest of the Secrets and find the ones that help you the most. Add them to the basics.

Third: As soon as you can, establish a mission, a long-term purpose for your life. If you work hard to achieve your goals, most everything else will follow easily.

Fourth: Smile and laugh often and see what happens: happiness!

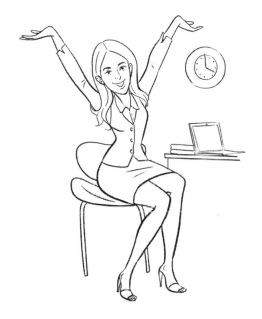

I am Living a *Happy, Healthy, Sexy, Long Life!*

Appendix

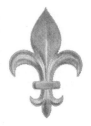

Acknowledgements/Reference By Secret

Experts, Researchers, Writers, Research Centers, Publications,
Journals, Universities, Medical Centers as credited or quoted

Secret #6 Restful Sleep
- Prevention Magazine
- Robert Duvall, Actor

Secret #8 The Benefits of Laughing Out Loud
- Mark Twain/ Samuel Langhorne Clemens
- Pundit, author, humorist

Secret #9 Ways to Make You Laugh
- Mary Oliver, poet

Secret #10 Smile, Smile Often and See What Happens
- e.e cummings, poet, playwright, author essayist

His Holiness the Fourteenth Dalai lama

Secret # 15 Romanticize Your Goals
- The Play: The Man of La Mancha
- Mitch Leigh, composer
- Joe Darion, songwriter
- Peter O'/Toole, actor, singer

Secret #16 Take Control of Your Balance
- Jen Magro, exercise trainer

Secret #17 Improve Your Balance With Exercise
- Mayo Clinic
- Mike Ross, Exercise Physiologist and Author
- The Balance Manual

Secret #18 Stress and Boredom
- Rex Huppke, Columnist
- Gloria Mark, Professor, University of California

Secret #19 Handling Stress
- John Keats, poet

Secret #37 Zollipops
- Alina Moore
- 9 Year old inventor
- Tom Moore
- Alina's Father, Product Consultant

Secret #38 A New Spin on Potatoes
- Institute of Medicine
- WIC, Women's, Infants' and Children's Program

Secret #39 The Vigor of Vitamins
- Harvard T.H. Chan School of Public Health

Secret #42 The Meditterannean Diet
- Yian Gu
- Assistant Professor of Neuropsychology at Columbia University

Secret #43 The Versatility of Coconuts
- The Coconut Research Center

Secret #46 Prepare For Your Run, and Run Right
- Patrick Murphy
- Physical/Exercise Trainer
- Personal Best Fitness and Training Program

Secret #47 The Draw and the Dangers of Treadmill Running
- Sports and Fitness Industry Association
- Mike Bracho
- Physiologist, Calgary, Alberta, Canada

Secret # 50 Select Spa Therapies That Are Best For You
- Journal of the American Medical Association

Secret #54 The Art of Non-Sexual Touching and Hugs
- Virginia Satir
- 20th Century Family Therapist
- Bonnie Beaver
- Professor of Animal Behavior, College of Veterinary Medicine Texas A&M

Secret #56 Build a Roster of Diverse Friendships
- Dr. Suzy Green
- Clinical Coaching Psychologist & Founder of the Positive Institute
- Dominique Berlucci
- Life Coach and Author of "The Happiness Code"

Secret #71 A Daily Goblet of Red Wine
- Neurosychiatric Disease/Treatment Journal
- Harvard University
- The Hunt Study, Norway
- Journal of Biological Research. By Researchers and Purdue University

Secret #72 The Case for White Wine
- Researchers. The Universities of Connecticut and Milan
- Deborah Gavito.
- Director of the Counter Vegetable Bistro and Organic Bar in New York City
- A.M. Authority Nutrition

Secret #77 Just One Cup of Coffee
- The Italian Longitudinal Study

Secret #78 The Rewards of a Pursuit With a Purpose
- Deepak Chopra
  Founder, Chopra Center for Wellness

Secret #79 The Importance of a Purpose In Retirement
- AARP Magazine
- Benjamin Franklin
- Diplomat, author, statesman, publisher

Secret #83 Enjoy Unconditional Love
- Henry David Thoreau
- Poet, Naturalist

Secret #84 Live Your Passing Years Raucously
- Regina Barreca
- English Professor, University of Connecticut

Secret #87 Telomeres, A Key to Aging Well
- Dr. Richard Cawthon
- Genetic Research at The University of Utah

Secret #88 Move Slowly When You Make a Change in Your Life
- William Shakespeare
- Playwright
- Johann Wolfgang von Goethe
- German Philosopher

Other Works By Victoria D. Schmidt

Available on victoriadschmidt.com

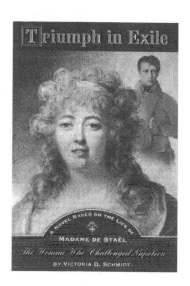

Triumph in Exile
A novel based on the life of Madame de Staël
the woman who challenged Napoleon

Germaine de Staël was not a beautiful woman.

Yet she captured the imagination and won the love of some of the most powerful men at the heart of the French Revolution and the era that followed. One colossus, however refused to fall under her spell--and she took him on as an adversary. He was Napoleon Bonaparte.

Triumph in Exile is a fictionalized chronicle of Germaine de Staël's life, based on historical fact, which focuses on her confrontation with Napoleon as well as her many tempestuous love affairs... some with gallant men much younger than she. Victoria D. Schmidt vividly tells the story of a towering woman, who motivated by uncompromising principles and fortified with unlimited resources from her father, helped to bring down an unbridled tyrant and altered the course of history in France-and without exaggeration to say -- the rest of the world.

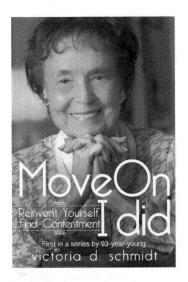

Move On! Reinvent Yourself! Find Contentment! I Did!

Victoria Dabrowski Schmidt lives a full life. She flourished in the light of an adoring husband. raised a loving daughter and continues to achieve prominence and acclaim in her career. After a fifty-eight year marriage she lost her husband to Parkinson's disease, reinvented herself and has found contentment. When her husband died. Victoria found several havens including scores of publications that helped her as she grieved and gave her a sense of peace.

However. she felt there was a need. a single volume with a wide range of resources. people. places and websites. and more where those with losses can find solace and gratifying new life options. She undertook the task herself. The result is **Move On! Reinvent Yourself. Find Contentment. I Did!**

Move On! I Did! is an upbeat book about love. loss and hope. It is positive. with a "to do" list for when you are not sure what to do next. You will find a "feel better" guide you can turn to after a major loss. a devastating experience or just a typical bad day. Uplifting. engaging and enlightening, this book is practical. informative and educational. Its message opens doors to "good life options" and cheers you on to rise up and **Move On!**

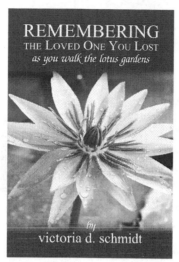

Remembering the Loved One You Lost.

A companion piece to Move on! Reinvent Yourself! Find Contentment! I did!, is a little book with a big, caring heart. The passages with images of the noble lotus in this inspirational volume will help those who have lost loving partners find solace, comfort, and peace. Many of the lines of poetry also reach out to console those who are grieving for dear friends or other family members who have left them in sorrow. Dying is not the end, it is a part of life, a beginning of contemplative thought and a reminder of the wonders of living.

About the Author

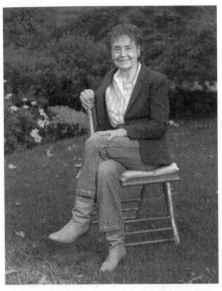

Victoria Dabrowski Schmidt is a woman who has lived, loved and worked an admirable life through nine decades ... and continues to do so. Her wit and style are timeless, as are her energy and curiosity. She has a thirst for knowledge that keeps her current despite her years. She has had it all without ever considering the alternative ... love, family, work and friends. She dreams big and has passion and a willing spirit to share the successes and failures that make her such an inspiration.

Victoria climbed the ladder of success by way of being a fashion editor at **Woman's Day** magazine in New York City, serving as the Director of Travel and Tourism for New Jersey under Governor Thom Kean, running her own successful advertising and public relations firm in Newark and Bernardsville, New Jersey and founding an ESL business in Poland the land of her heritage. Early in her career, she took to pen with **Triumph in Exile**, a book celebrating a woman who had a strong voice and made a difference, a topic that would stay with Victoria.

After fifty-eight years in a happy, loving marriage, author Victoria D. Schmidt lost her husband Ralph to Parkinson's disease. She was inspired by the loss to write Move On! Reinvent Yourself! Find Contentment! I Did! and Remembering The Loved One You Lost. Victoria again honors her husband in her dedication to him for her current book, Victoria's 95 Secrets.

The author has been recognized for her accomplishments throughout her career with countless awards. Most recently, just after her 95th birthday, she was one of four recipients of the 2016, 35th Annual Women of Achievement Award sponsored by the New Jersey State Federation of Women's Clubs.

Victoria lives in rural Oldwick, New Jersey with Dominique, her gentle whippet.